PRINCIPLES OF BIOLOGICAL CONTROL

PRINCIPLES
OF BIOLOGICAL
CONTROL

by
David F. Horrobin
MA, DPhil, BM, BCh.

Professor of Medical Physiology,
University College, Nairobi.
Scholar of Balliol College and
late Fellow of Magdalen College,
Oxford.

MTP
Medical and Technical Publishing Co. Ltd., Chiltern House, Aylesbury.

Published in Great Britain in 1970
by MTP, Medical and Technical Publishing
Co. Ltd., Chiltern House, Aylesbury, Bucks.
Copyright © D. F. Horrobin 1970
Softcover reprint of the hardcover 1st edition 1970

ISBN-13: 978-94-011-7128-1   e-ISBN-13: 978-94-011-7126-7
DOI: 10.1007/978-94-011-7126-7

Contents

Contents

Illustrations

Principles of biological control

17 Schematic outline of the factors which may influence the function of the arterial blood pressure receptors. The receptors may be stretched either by a rise of the blood pressure inside the vessel or by contraction of the muscle fibres in the wall. If the fibrous tissue of the vessel wall becomes stiffer, a higher blood pressure will be required to produce the same degree of receptor stretch.

Preface

The study of the normal function of the animal and human organisms and of the diseases which disturb that normal function is largely the study of control mechanisms. These control mechanisms are essential for the survival of an organism in a more or less hostile environment. In many ways they clearly resemble the control mechanisms devised by electronic engineers for running machinery of all kinds and there are many remarkable parallels between biology and engineering.

However, it should not be forgotten that the biological systems were on the scene first and that the engineering is a parallel and independent development. It is therefore perhaps a pity that in recent years the study of biological control systems has tended to be dominated by mathematicians and engineers who have moved from these more precise disciplines into biology. As a consequence of this dominance, one often gets the impression that the principles of biological control can be understood only after one has undergone a rather high-powered course in electronic control theory. It often seems to be assumed that it is electronics which must do all the teaching while biology and medicine must do all the learning. In fact I suspect that biological control mechanisms are considerably more sophisticated than anything yet available in the world of the physical sciences and that in the long run biology will teach more to control engineers than vice versa.

The preponderance of physically and mathematically trained individuals in the field of biological control mechanisms has led to a dearth of writing that is intelligible to students, and even to research workers, in biology and medicine. Few of those who approach biology from the viewpoint of the physical sciences realise how mathematically unsophisticated most biologists are or how frightened they are of apparently complex equations. Few also realise how very rarely is it that a

Principles of biological control

knowledge of mathematics is of any importance in biological research. Many biological and medical tests contain a brief and excessively elementary account of control theory as illustrated by the simplest of simple household thermostats. But above this level, most accounts of biological control wade deeper and deeper into what many biologists regard as the mire of mathematical complexity. There is virtually nothing in between the elementary and the complex and as a result few biologists know anything about control theory. This is a great pity for a completely non-mathematical understanding of the principles of design of any good control system can illumine biological mechanisms and can be a useful guide to further research.

This brief book is therefore an unashamedly mathematics and jargon-free guide to the principles of control as seen by someone with a strongly biological viewpoint. I hope that it may fill a gap between the sketchy textbook accounts and the complex treatises. It was originally written for undergraduates in the biological sciences, particularly those studying medicine, physiology, zoology and psychology. However, in manuscript form it has been read by two other quite different groups of people, university lecturers in biology and senior school pupils. In both cases I was surprised by the enthusiasm of the response. The university lecturers felt that this account of biological control shed new light on their work and gave them new ideas for research. The school pupils realised for the first time that biology was a genuinely dynamic subject with greater possibilities than they had imagined. Therefore although the book is written primarily for undergraduates I hope it will not be entirely scorned by more senior biologists and doctors and that it may be placed in many school libraries where it may stimulate younger students to see the interest and possibilities of biology. The introduction is so written that it can be understood by those with very little knowledge of biology or of science. The more senior reader should therefore skip the introductory section.

DAVID F. HORROBIN   December, 1969.
Nairobi, Kenya.

Chapter 1

Introduction

For the animal organism the central problem of existence is that of maintaining the stability of its structure and function in the face of constant internal and external assaults. Externally the body may be assaulted most obviously by extremes of environmental temperature. Internally it is assaulted among other things by the continual production of the waste products of its own function. The core of the body's problem is that especially in warm-blooded organisms, the cells can function normally only if the fluid in which they are all bathed is maintained at a more or less constant temperature and at a constant chemical composition. If this maintenance fails and if the temperature and chemical composition vary outside very narrowly defined limits, the delicate biochemical reactions which go on within the cells may be severely disrupted. The consequences are death of the cells and ultimately of the whole organism.

The requirements of cells are many and complex. Only the most important will be briefly mentioned here. The functioning of the cell depends on energy which is largely supplied by the breakdown of fats and carbohydrates (particularly glucose). This energy can be released in adequate quantities only if ample oxygen is available. The consumption of food materials and oxygen leads to the production of carbon dioxide and other waste materials which must be removed from the environment of the cell if they are not to cause poisoning. In addition to the major and well-known factors just mentioned, normal cell function requires that the fluid bathing the cells should

1

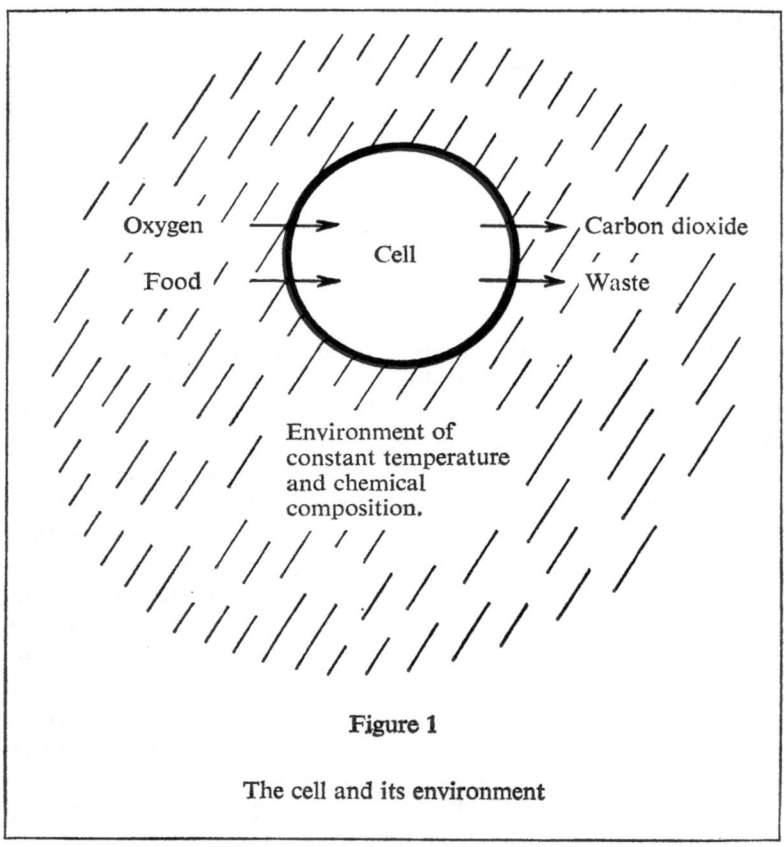

Figure 1

The cell and its environment

contain the right concentrations of almost innumerable other substances such as sodium, potassium, calcium and bicarbonate ions and many different hormones such as cortisol produced by the adrenal cortex and thyroid hormone produced by the thyroid gland.

In order to maintain constant temperature and chemical composition of the fluid surrounding the cells, many supporting organs and systems are required. Perhaps the central one of

2

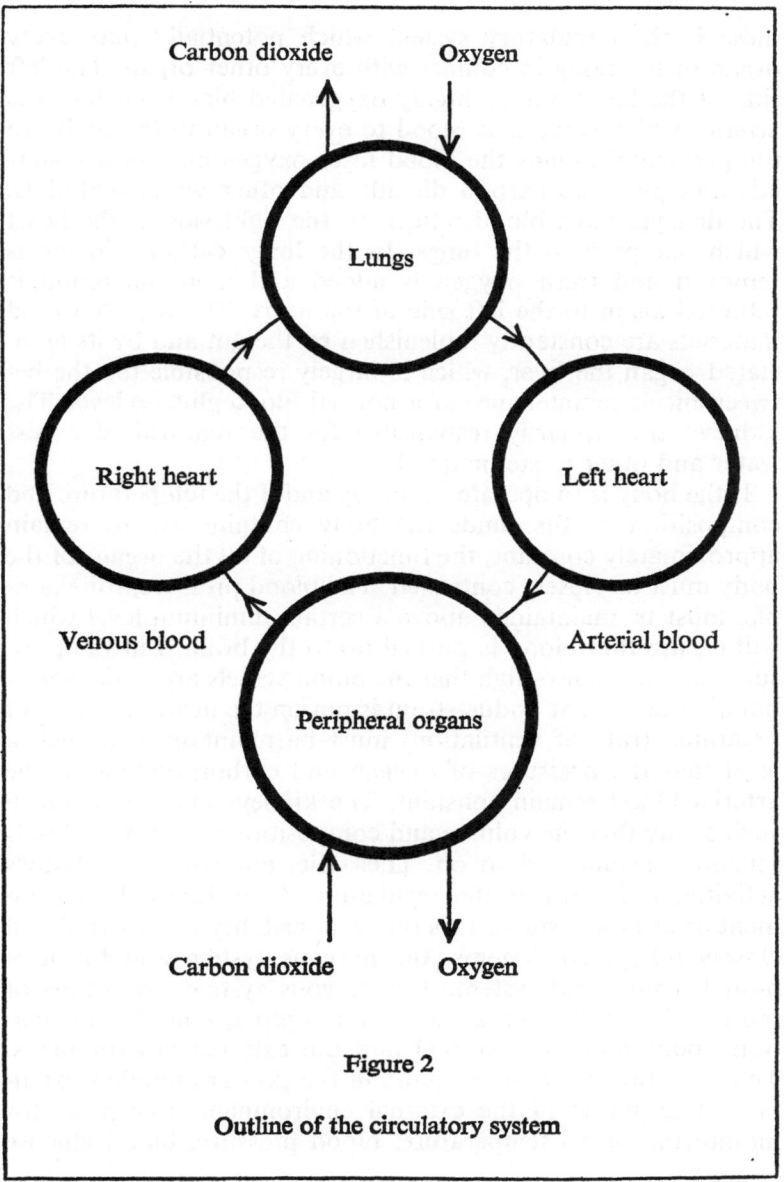

Figure 2

Outline of the circulatory system

these is the circulatory system which potentially puts every organ in the body in contact with every other organ. The left side of the heart pumps highly oxygenated blood out into the arteries which carry that blood to every organ in the body. In the peripheral organs the blood loses oxygen and food materials and picks up carbon dioxide and other waste materials. The deoxygenated blood returns to the right side of the heart which pumps it to the lungs. In the lungs carbon dioxide is removed and fresh oxygen is added and then the blood is returned again to the left side of the heart. The depleted food materials are constantly replenished by the gut and by its associated organ the liver, which is largely responsible for the between meals maintenance of a normal blood glucose level. The kidneys are primarily responsible for the removal of excess water and other waste material.

If the body is to operate smoothly and if the temperature and composition of the fluids the body contains are to remain approximately constant, the functioning of all the organs of the body must be closely controlled. The blood pressure, for example, must be maintained above a certain minimum level which will ensure that blood is pushed up to the brain. But the pressure must not go so high that the blood vessels are in danger of bursting or so that undue strain is put on the heart. The rate of breathing (rate of ventilation) must be maintained at such a level that the pressures of oxygen and carbon dioxide in the arterial blood remain constant. The kidneys must function in such a way that the volume and composition of the body fluids remain constant and so on. This strict control of the body's activities is known as the regulation of the internal environment or as homeostasis. It is the responsibility of two vital and closely integrated systems, the nervous system and the hormonal (endocrine) system. The nervous system, by means of sensing devices known as sensory receptors, collects information about both the internal and the external environments. The eyes, the ears and receptors in the skin are familiar examples of monitors of the external environment. Receptors for monitoring blood temperature, blood pressure, blood glucose

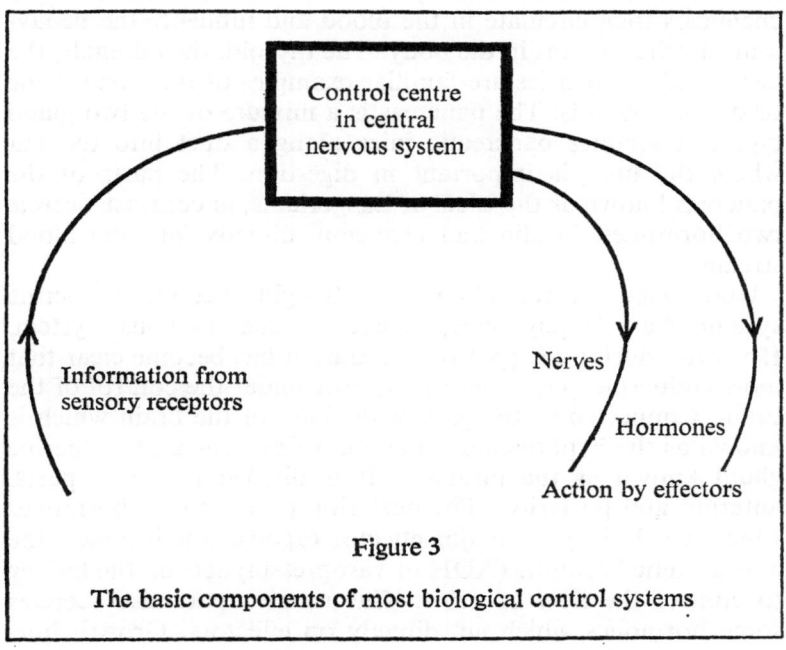

Figure 3

The basic components of most biological control systems

concentration, joint position and the state of contraction of muscles are but a few examples of receptors collecting information about the internal environment. All this information is carried to the central nervous system (the brain and spinal cord) in the form of impulses in sensory nerves. In the brain are control centres which continually assess the significance of the information they receive. They then send out appropriate instructions along motor or effector nerves to the organs (effectors) which are responsible for maintaining the constancy of the internal environment.

In several parts of the body there are glands which secrete fluid materials along ducts. The salivary glands which secrete saliva into the mouth and the sweat glands which secrete sweat on to the skin are good examples. But there are also other glands which do not have ducts and which secrete chemicals

5

known as hormones directly into the blood stream. These chemicals then circulate in the blood and influence the behaviour of other organs in the body The thyroid, the adrenals, the testes and the ovaries are familiar examples of these endocrine or ductless glands. The pancreas is a mixture of the two gland types. It secretes pancreatic juice along a duct into the gut where the juice is important in digestion. The parts of the pancreas known as the islets of Langerhans, in contrast, secrete two hormones, insulin and glucagon, directly into the blood stream.

Until relatively recently it was thought that the endocrine system was largely independent of the nervous system. However, during the past two decades it has become clear that most endocrine glands act as effectors under the control of the brain. Connected to the part of the base of the brain which is known as the hypothalamus there is a tiny pea-sized endocrine gland known as the pituitary. It is divided into two parts, anterior and posterior. The posterior part secretes hormones which act directly on major effector organs. For instance, the anti-diuretic hormone (ADH or vasopressin) acts on the kidney to control the flow of urine. The anterior part also secretes some hormones which act directly on effectors. Growth hormone (somatotrophin) helps to control the blood glucose level and the rate of growth while prolactin (LTH or luteotrophic hormone) stimulates the breasts to secrete milk. But the anterior pituitary also secretes several other hormones which act not directly on effectors but on other endocrine glands. Thyrotrophic hormone (TSH or thyroid-stimulating hormone) controls the output of thyroid hormone from the thyroid gland. Adrenocorticotrophic hormone (ACTH) controls the output of cortisol from the adrenal gland. The gonadotrophic hormones stimulate the production of sex hormones from the ovaries in the female and the testes in the male. These major endocrine glands thus seem to be governed by the anterior pituitary which has often been called "the conductor of the endocrine orchestra".

The anterior pituitary has an unusual blood supply. The

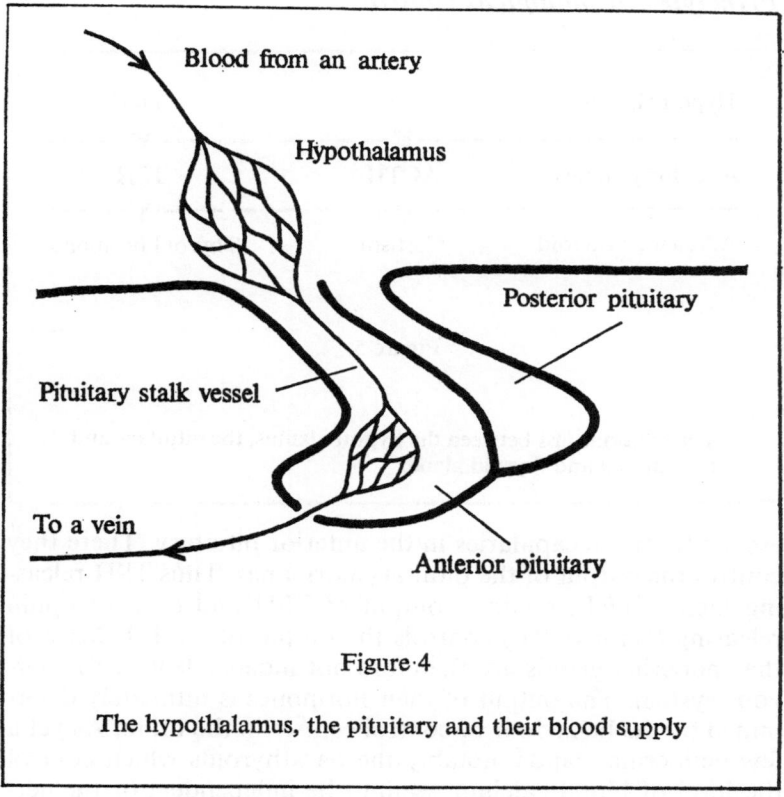

Figure·4

The hypothalamus, the pituitary and their blood supply

blood vessels to the hypothalamus break up into the minute tubes known as capillaries. These capillaries then join up into larger vessels, but instead of pouring their blood into veins and so back to the heart, these larger vessels travel down the pituitary stalk and break up again to form another set of capillaries in the anterior pituitary. It is now known that the nerve cells of the hypothalamus secrete into the blood capillaries substances known as releasing factors. There seems to be a separate releasing factor for each of the anterior pituitary hormones. These releasing factors travel in the blood down the stalk and then

7

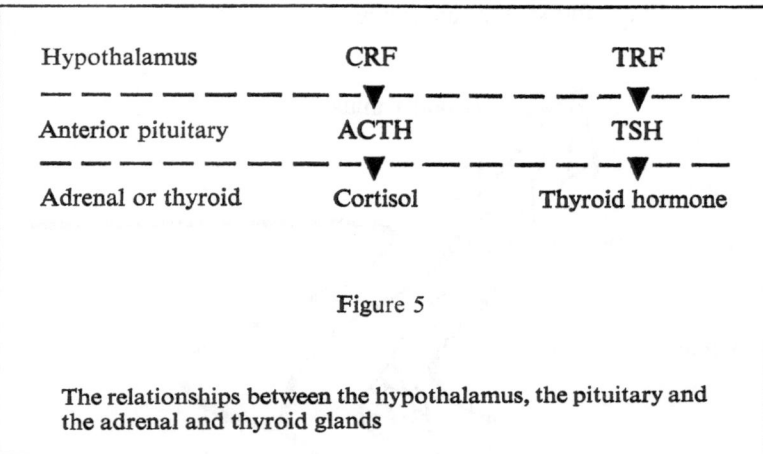

Figure 5

The relationships between the hypothalamus, the pituitary and the adrenal and thyroid glands

escape from the capillaries in the anterior pituitary. There they control the output of the pituitary hormones. Thus TSH releasing factor (TRF) controls output of TSH and corticotrophin releasing factor (CRF) controls the output of ACTH. Most of the endocrine glands are therefore not independent of the nervous system. The output of their hormones is ultimately determined by the behaviour of control centres in the brain. As yet a few endocrine glands, notably the parathyroids which control the level of blood calcium, seem to be independent of the nervous system. A final decision as to whether they are truly entirely free of its influence must await further research.

And so the behaviour of the organs of the body can be seen to depend largely on the control exercised over them by the nervous and endocrine systems. The remainder of this book is concerned with describing the principles on which these control systems operate.

Chapter 2

Basic principles of control

The fundamental components which a control system of any type must possess can be clearly seen in the design of a simple household thermostat which controls the temperature of a room in a cold climate. The thermostat has three essential components, a thermometer, a source of heat, and a switch for turning the heat source on and off. The thermometer is linked to the switch and the two are so designed that whenever the temperature of the room falls below a certain level, the heat source is switched on. Whenever the temperature rises above that level the heating is switched off. The cycle of events is repeated again and again as the temperature of the room oscillates around its set level, being pushed up by the heating system and pulled down by the cold outside environment. This oscillation about a fixed point is sometimes known as *"hunting"*.

The magnitude of the swings in the temperature of the room depends on two things, the sensitivity of the thermometer and switching system and the delicacy of the control of the heat source. If the thermometer turns on the switch when the temperature falls only a fraction of a degree below the set level, X, and if the heating is turned up only gently so that the temperature does not rise very rapidly and overshoot X, the magnitude of the oscillations will be small. On the other hand, if the thermometer operates the switch only when the temperature has fallen several degrees below X and if the heat source is very powerful and poorly regulated, the temperature, while remaining centred on X may oscillate over a wide range.

Principles of biological control

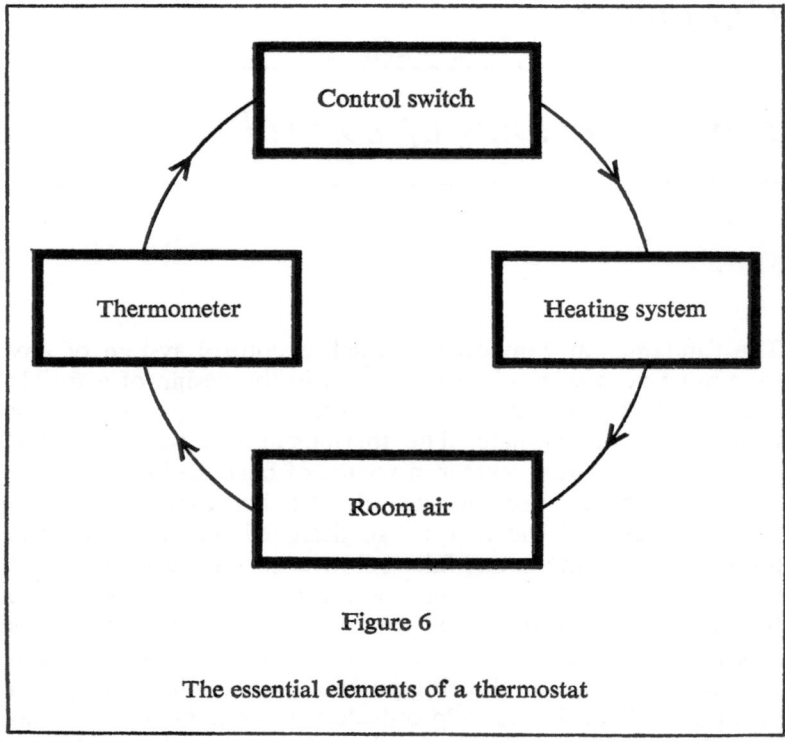

Figure 6

The essential elements of a thermostat

Most thermostats have at least one other component and that is a device whereby the set level may be altered. There is usually a knob which can modify the behaviour of the switch so that instead of maintaining the temperature close to X, it maintains it close to Y. The heat source is turned on and off at a room temperature in the vicinity of Y instead of one in the vicinity of X.

A point worth noting about the thermostat and one which applies to most physical and biological control systems is the siting of the sensing device, in this case the thermometer. The device is not placed at a point where it can measure the intensity of the forces tending to disturb the system. If the thermometer were to do that, it would have to be placed on the outside wall where it could measure the temperature of the outside environment and thus the intensity of the cold with which the heating system had to cope. In practice, sensing devices which measure the intensity of the forces tending to disturb a system have been found inadequate for accurate control. In the remainder of this book such devices will be called *disturbance detectors*. As an experiment, the thermometer of a thermostat can be put outside the house whose internal temperature is to be controlled. It can be linked to the heating system so that the colder the outside environment becomes, the more heating is turned on. If such a system is tried it is found that the temperature inside the house fluctuates wildly and the result is most unsatisfactory. The system fails primarily because there is no simple direct relationship between the environmental temperature and the temperature inside the house.

In any real house there is constant interference from uncontrollable variations in the rate of heat production and heat loss. People produce heat and the more people there are in the house, the greater will be the heat production. A thermometer on the outside wall could not cater for this. People also open and close curtains and windows and doors thus altering the rate of heat loss. Again a thermometer on the outside wall which simply measures the environmental temperature cannot take these factors, which have important effects on the internal temperature, into consideration. The control system is therefore certain to fail.

This means that in any good control system the sensing device should measure not the magnitude of a particular disturbing force. Instead it should measure the result of the interaction between the stress which is tending to disturb the status quo and the factors which are tending to maintain the steady state. This means that it should monitor the state of the factor whose constancy is desired. Therefore in a good thermostat the thermometer is put inside the room whose temperature is to be kept constant and not on the outside wall of that room. The temperature inside the room is the resultant of all the

Principles of biological control

factors influencing heat production in the room and the heat loss from it. The magnitude and behaviour of each individual factor do not need to be understood for the system to work. It is sufficient for the thermometer simply to measure the temperature of the room which is the result of the interaction of all the various factors. The thermometer reading depends on the balance between all the factors causing heat production and all the ones promoting heat loss. Ideally at the desired temperature, heat loss just balances heat production. If heat production rises this is detected by the thermometer and the heating is turned down. If heat loss increases, the temperature falls, this is again detected by the thermometer and the heating is turned up. Such sensing devices in control systems are therefore sometimes known as *misalignment detectors* because they detect any deviation from the desired value which may result from an imbalance of the forces acting upon the factor which is being controlled.

Although it may seem superfluous to say so, it is essential to remember that in a good control system the factor which is being controlled is the one which remains constant in value. If the system is disturbed in any way, it is the factor which counteracts the disturbance which fluctuates. The level of the factor which is being controlled should not alter. In the thermostat example, if the system is a good one, the reading of the thermometer will remain constant no matter what the cold stress may be. It is the output of the heating system which will vary in order to cope with the varying intensity of the cold stress. But although the heat output varies while the thermometer reading remains constant, this does not mean that there is no connection between the two. Some people so misunderstand control systems that they believe that if the heating part of a thermostatic control device is functioning at a very high level then the thermometer reading must also be way off the desired mark in order to provide the necessary intense stimulus for such a big response. This very elementary point is so important and has so often been thoroughly misunderstood by biologists that it is worth describing in a very simple way the sequence of events which occurs in a household thermostat when the temperature of the outside air steadily becomes colder.

1. The cold stress exceeds the existing heat output and the temperature of the room falls slightly.

2. The fall in temperature is detected by the thermometer and in order to restore the balance between heat loss and heat production the power of the heating system is turned up by the control mechanism.

3. The temperature of the room returns to the desired level.

4. If the cold stress continues to increase, again the balance between heat loss and heat production will be upset. The thermometer reading will fall, heat output will be further increased and the temperature will again get back to its set level.

5. If the outside temperature falls further, the cycle may be repeated many times. Eventually the heating system will be roaring full blast but the room temperature will remain what it was before the cold stress began. This situation is a consequence of the fact that the thermometer is acting as a misalignment detector and not a disturbance detector. It simply measures the result of the interaction between heat loss and heat production. As the environmental temperature falls, the heating system is turned up correspondingly.

There are several instances in biology where research workers have failed to understand that a massive effector response does not have to be produced by a large deviation from the normal level of the factor which is supposed to be kept constant. A classic example was a violent controversy not so many years ago about the mechanism by which the rate of ventilation (breathing) is increased in mild to moderate exercise. It had long been known that there are sensitive receptors for measuring the concentration of carbon dioxide in arterial blood. If the arterial carbon dioxide level rises the information is sent to the brain where the control centre orders an increase in the ventilation rate. The faster rate of breathing then gets rid of the carbon dioxide more rapidly. Under normal circumstances the receptors act as misalignment detectors: carbon dioxide enters

Principles of biological control

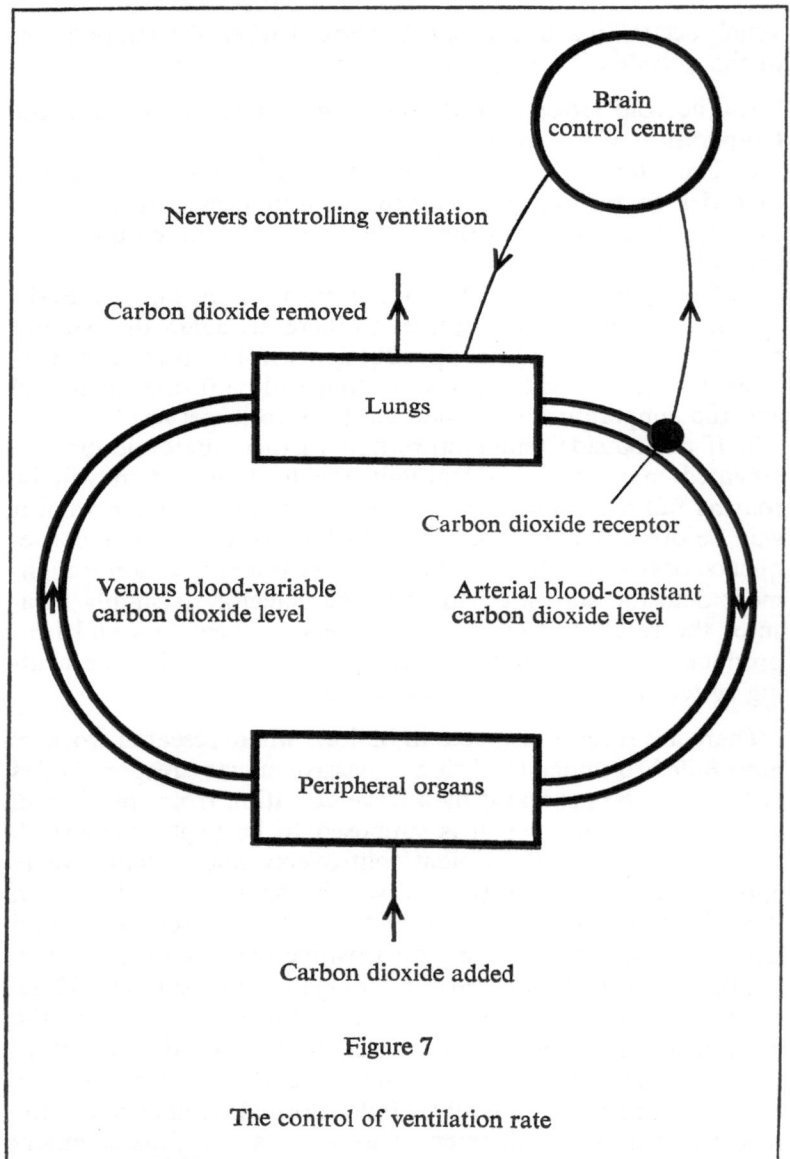

Figure 7

The control of ventilation rate

the blood in the capillaries and the carbon dioxide-rich blood passes via the veins to the heart. But only after the blood has been passed through the lungs where the carbon dioxide is normally removed is the carbon dioxide level measured. The receptors measure the result of the interaction between the action of the peripheral organs in adding carbon dioxide to the blood and the action of the lungs in removing it. Only if there is an imbalance is the ventilation rate changed.

The increase in ventilation rate in exercise can therefore be relatively simply explained as follows:

1. The exercising muscles produce large amounts of carbon dioxide which raise the carbon dioxide content of the venous blood above normal.

2. At the resting rate of ventilation, the excess of carbon dioxide is not all removed during the passage through the lungs and so the carbon dioxide in the arterial blood rises.

3. This increase is detected by the arterial receptors. The information is sent to the brain and the control centres in the brain increase the ventilation rate in order to cope with the increased rate of carbon dioxide production. The arterial carbon dioxide level returns to normal. Nevertheless it is the arterial carbon dioxide receptors which have brought about the increased ventilation rate, even though as the result of the operation of the control system the arterial carbon dioxide level is held approximately constant.

But some physiologists failed to see this. They reasoned that since the arterial carbon dioxide level does not rise in moderate exercise, the increase in ventilation could not be brought about by the functioning of the arterial carbon dioxide receptors. Many elaborate experiments were carried out in the effort to find other factors which could stimulate ventilation. Only recently has it been understood that the fact that the arterial carbon dioxide level remains constant is the very best argument for the importance of carbon dioxide in controlling ventilation in exercise. In contrast, if the arterial carbon dioxide level were to fluctuate considerably one might then suspect that the changes in ventilation were unrelated to the arterial carbon dioxide level. Then one might start looking seriously for other factors.

Chapter 3

Negative and positive feedback

A feedback mechanism is said to exist when a change in a system leads to a sequence of events whose end result is to produce another change in the same system. That may sound complex but a few examples will make it clear.

There are two main types of feedback, negative and positive. The former is by far the most common in biological situations. With negative feedback, if a system is disturbed that disturbance sets in motion a train of events which counteract the disturbance and tend to restore the system to its original state. The negative feedback principle has therefore been called the law of sheer cussedness because the mechanism resists any attempts to change the system: negative feedback mechanisms therefore tend to act in favour of stability. As might be expected from its name, positive feedback is quite different. In this case a disturbance in a system sets in motion a train of events which increases the disturbance still further. Positive feedback mechanisms therefore lead to instability and are rare in biology.

The thermostat is an excellent non-biological example of a negative feedback mechanism. If the temperature falls, the change is detected by the thermometer and a sequence of events is set in motion to return the temperature to its set value. Because the end result of the operation of a negative feedback mechanism is stability, it is not surprising that there are innumerable biological examples of such mechanisms. The body's own temperature control system is one. If the body temperature rises, the change is detected by receptors which sample the arterial blood. The information is sent to the control system in the brain and this sets in motion mechanisms aimed at increasing the rate of heat loss. The rate of blood flow to the skin is greatly increased, so carrying heat from the deep organs to the surface where it can be lost to the surrounding environment. Sweat is secreted on to the skin surface and as it evaporates the skin is cooled. On the other hand if the body temperature falls, the rate of skin blood flow is reduced and shivering may be started in order to increase heat production. In both cases a change in body temperature leads to events which reverse that change and restore the system to normal.

The control of the carbon dioxide level of arterial blood is another good example which has already been discussed. If the carbon dioxide level rises as the result of exercise, this is detected by the arterial receptors. The information is conveyed to the brain and the ventilation rate is increased to get rid of the carbon dioxide excess. If the carbon dioxide level falls, then the rate of ventilation also falls and carbon dioxide accumulates until it reaches its normal level.

The output of hormones from most of the endocrine glands is also controlled by negative feedback mechanisms. The adrenal cortex will serve as an example. One of the most important hormones which it produces is known as cortisol (hydrocortisone). The rate of production of cortisol is determined by the blood level of ACTH which is secreted by the anterior pituitary. The rate of production of ACTH is determined by the amount of CRF passing down the pituitary stalk vessels from the hypothalamus. And the output of CRF is determined by the level of cortisol in the blood reaching the hypothalamus. The hypothalamus sets the desired level of cortisol in the blood. If the cortisol concentration rises above this the outputs of CRF and ACTH and hence of cortisol are reduced. If the cortisol concentration falls below the desired level, CRF, ACTH and therefore cortisol outputs are increased. The mechanism therefore tends to maintain the cortisol concentration constant.

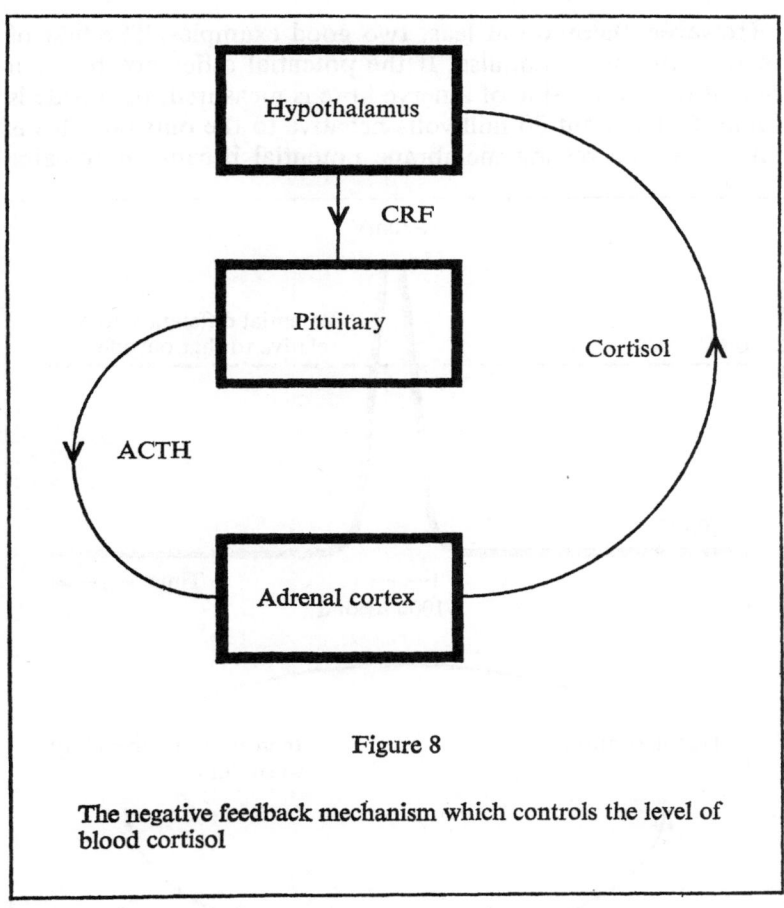

Figure 8

The negative feedback mechanism which controls the level of blood cortisol

With positive feedback, a disturbance leads to events which further increase the disturbance. This increased disturbance activates the positive feedback mechanism still more and so the state of the system changes very rapidly indeed. The positive feedback principle is perhaps more familiarly known as the vicious circle. Positive feedback mechanisms are unstable and are therefore rare in biology.

19

Principles of biological control

However, there are at least two good examples. The first of these is the nerve impulse. If the potential difference between the inside and outside of a nerve fibre is measured, the inside is found to be about 70 millivolts negative to the outside. This is known as the resting membrane potential because it remains

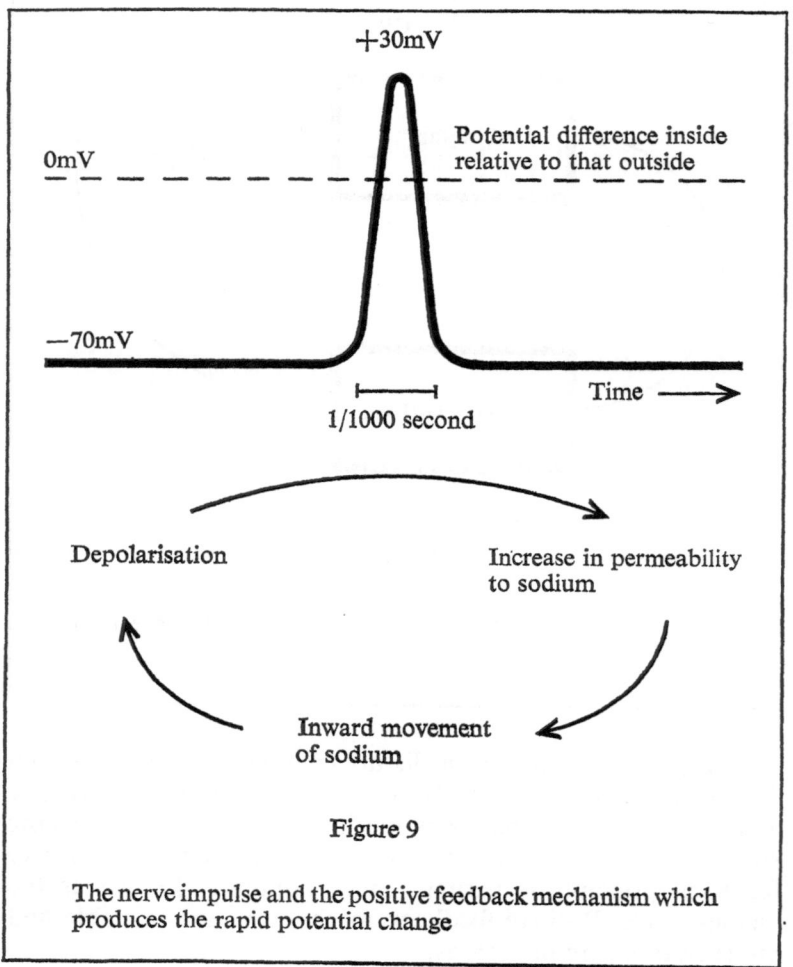

Figure 9

The nerve impulse and the positive feedback mechanism which produces the rapid potential change

steady as long as the nerve is inactive. Before the positive feedback mechanism can be understood, two other facts must be known: these are that the resting membrane is effectively impermeable to sodium ions and that the concentration of sodium ions in the fluid outside the fibre is very much greater than the concentration in the fluid inside the fibre. There is therefore a large concentration gradient which would push sodium rapidly into the fibre if the membrane were permeable to it. If an electric shock is given to the nerve fibre, a nerve impulse may be initiated by the following sequence of events:

1. The shock reduces the potential difference between the inside and outside of the fibre. It is said to depolarise the fibre.

2. This depolarisation makes the nerve fibre membrane slightly permeable to sodium. Sodium ions therefore move into the fibre down their concentration gradient.

3. Since the sodium ions are positively charged, their inward movement further reduces the internal negativity of the fibre.

4. This further depolarisation increases the permeability to sodium still more. Sodium ions rush in even more rapidly, this produces a further depolarisation and so on.

5. Eventually sodium rushes in so rapidly that the inside of the nerve fibre actually becomes positive to the outside. The movement stops only when the concentration gradient pushing sodium in is balanced by the electrical force pushing sodium out. (Like charges repel one another, and once the inside of the fibre becomes positive it will tend to repel the positively charged sodium ions.)

However, if the membrane were to remain positively charged inside, the nerve would be inexcitable and could conduct no further impulses. There is therefore a cut off point. For reasons which are as yet poorly understood, after about one-thousandth of a second the membrane again becomes effectively impermeable to sodium. The membrane potential returns to its original level and the sodium ions are pumped out of the fibre. This demonstrates that positive feedback systems can be tolerated in biology only if at some point there is a cut out which breaks the cycle and returns the system to its former state. If this were not so, the positive feedback system could operate once only and that would not be much use to any animal.

The other example of positive feedback is much less well known and is still the subject of intensive research. In female mammals, the release of eggs from the ovary (ovulation) seems to be brought about by a sudden surge in the output of one of the gonadotrophic hormones, luteinising hormone (LH), from the anterior pituitary. The level of luteinising hormone both before and after ovulation is low, but at the time of ovulation there is a sudden and spectacular rise to a peak of hormone output followed by an almost equally rapid fall. In fact, the general shape of a graph showing LH output during the female sexual cycle does not look unlike the shape of an action potential. Whenever anything rises as dramatically as the output of LH at ovulation, it is wise to look for a positive feedback mechanism. This is especially true when the rapid rise is followed by a rapid fall indicating the operation of a cut out.

One of the actions of LH on the ovary is to stimulate the output of a hormone called progesterone. Progesterone is an unusual substance which seems to have a dual action on the nervous system. When the nervous system is exposed to progesterone following a period when progesterone has been absent, the first action of the hormone is to excite cells. But after a short time this excitatory effect wears off and the progesterone then depresses and inhibits nerve function. For some time before ovulation there is virtually no progesterone. Then, for reasons which are still obscure, just before ovulation some progesterone appears. This excites the hypothalamus and increases the output of luteinising hormone releasing factor (LRF). LRF goes down the pituitary stalk blood vessels and increases the output of LH. LH increases the secretion of progesterone by the ovary. The progesterone further excites the hypothalamus and the positive feedback cycle continues with the blood levels of both LH and progesterone rising rapidly. The cut off occurs when the excitatory effect of progesterone wears off and is replaced by its inhibitory effect. The output of

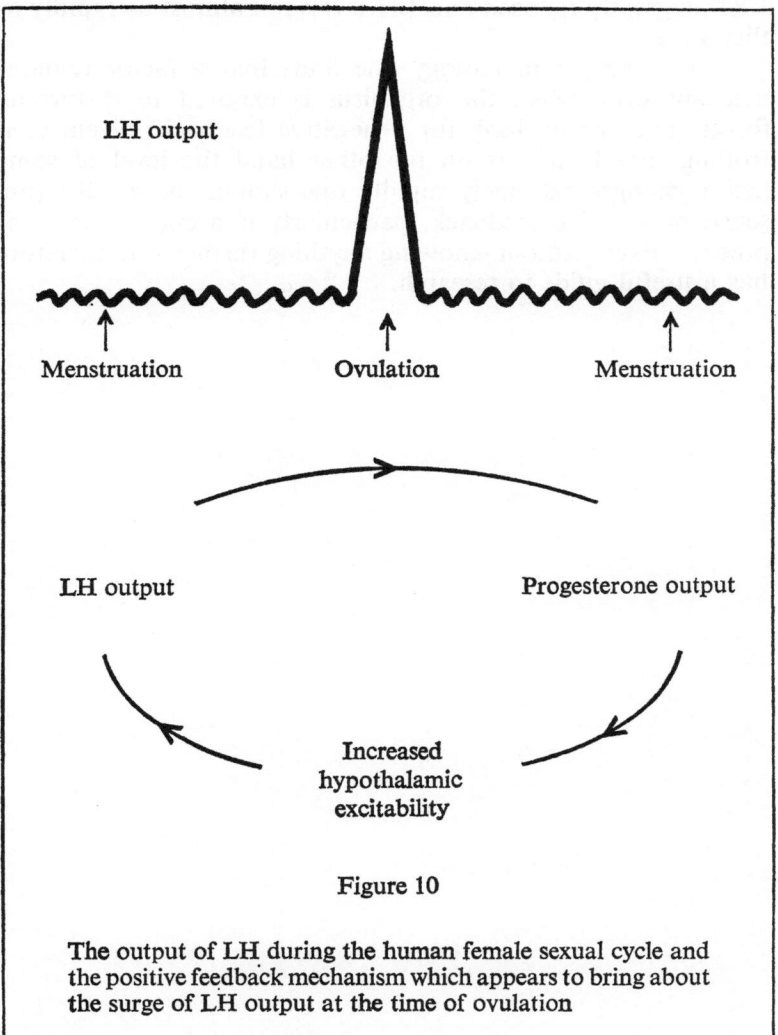

Figure 10

The output of LH during the human female sexual cycle and the positive feedback mechanism which appears to bring about the surge of LH output at the time of ovulation

23

Principles of biological control

LRF is greatly reduced and LH levels fall almost as rapidly as they rose.

In summary, if in biology one finds that a factor remains constant even when the organism is exposed to disturbing forces, one should look for a negative feedback system controlling that factor. If on the other hand the level of some factor changes extremely rapidly one should suspect the presence of positive feedback, particularly if a cut-off device is present. Even without knowing anything further one therefore has a useful guide to research.

Chapter 4

The value of disturbance detectors

It is a pity that most biological texts do not discuss control mechanisms of greater complexity than very simple thermostats. It is an even greater pity that when such more complex discussions are attempted the authors usually seem incapable of resisting the temptation to lapse into mathematics. Although it may be regrettable, authors should take note of the fact that most biologists and doctors are frightened of mathematics and automatically stop reading when they see some unfamiliar symbol. This is particularly sad because in discussions of biological control systems the mathematical treatment is often both incomplete and unnecessary. It seems to be put in to satisfy the needs of the author and not those of his readers. In consequence the readers, instead of grasping some points, albeit in a simple way, fail to grasp any at all. Therefore this and the following sections attempt to explain without the aid of mathematics and technical jargon some more complex aspects of control mechanisms. As will be seen, these concepts are of great importance and a lack of awareness of them ruins very many biological and medical experiments.

It was earlier pointed out that if a control mechanism is to work effectively it must be supplied with information by what is known as a misalignment detector. This picks up the discrepancy between the forces tending to push the system in one direction and those tending to push it in the other. It does not measure the intensity of the forces which are tending to disturb the system. Thus the thermometer of a household

Principles of biological control

thermostat is put not outside the house but in the room whose temperature is to be maintained at a steady level. There it measures the result of the interaction between the cold stress and the response of the heating system. Thus also carbon dioxide receptors are not put on the venous side of the circulatory system where they could measure the amount of excess carbon dioxide entering the blood from the peripheral tissues. Instead they are put on the arterial side where they monitor the result of the interaction between the entry of carbon dioxide into the blood in the tissues and its removal by the lungs. Long experience with physical control systems has demonstrated that systems which depend on misalignment detectors are stable while those which depend on disturbance detectors (detectors which measure the stress imposed on a system) are unstable and hopelessly unreliable.

However, although disturbance detectors are unsatisfactory when employed alone, there are many uses for them in both physical and biological control systems. If used in conjunction with misalignment detectors they can greatly increase the speed of response of a control mechanism. They can reduce the delay which inevitably occurs between a change in the system and the response to that change. For example, a thermostat could be made more effective if instead of a simple misalignment detector inside the house, there was in addition a disturbance detector on an outside wall. If the weather suddenly became cooler, this disturbance would be picked up by the outside thermometer before any alterations in the internal temperature could take place. If this information about the increased cold stress were then fed into the control system, the intensity of the heating could be gradually increased in anticipation of the expected fall in internal temperature. The information from the misalignment detector inside the house would then be used to make the final slight alterations in the heating system.

It is important that the disturbance detector should not dominate the control system. The final say in what happens to the intensity of heating should always depend on the misalignment detector. It is therefore clear that the control system should be so designed that it takes note only of *changes* in the behaviour of the disturbance detector. In the steady state, the information from the disturbance detector should be ignored. In contrast the heating should be controlled both by steady state and by changing information coming from the misalignment detector since the aim is to keep the reading of this detector constant. Furthermore, a disturbance detector should not produce too large an effector response: if it did, if the heating system were turned on full blast by a sudden fall in outside temperature, the temperature might well overswing and rise above the desired level. The link between the disturbance detector and the control system must be such that moderate effector changes in the right direction are produced, the final adjustment being dependent on information from the misalignment detector.

What would happen to such a thermostatic control system if one or other of the thermometers were destroyed? First consider the disturbance detector on the outside wall. Suppose that it is so arranged that the higher the outside temperature the more powerful is the signal it sends back to the control system. If the temperature falls the power of the signal will be reduced. If the disturbance detector suddenly stopped sending back information, the control system might therefore interpret this as a sudden fall in outside temperature and increase the output of the heating system. But within a short time the temperature inside the house would rise and the heating would be cut back to its original level as a result of the behaviour of the dominant internal misalignment detector. Loss of the outside thermometer would therefore produce no change in the temperature around which the system was being regulated and the internal temperature would still be relatively stable. In the steady state the temperature would be precisely the same as it would have been had the disturbance detector been functioning. The only difference will be in the nature of the response to changes in outside temperature. When the surroundings became colder, the heating system response will begin only when the change has produced a fall in internal temperature. The internal

27

Principles of biological control

temperature will therefore fall further before it can be counter-acted by an increased intensity of heating. Similarly if the environment becomes hotter the internal temperature will rise higher before the heating is turned down. Oscillations around the set temperature will therefore be wider than before.

The results will be quite different if the internal thermometer fails. The control system will interpret the sudden loss of information as a very rapid fall in internal temperature. The heating system will be turned up to its maximum level and since the control system is sensitive to the steady state discharge of the internal thermometer, this situation will continue even though the temperature inside the house rises rapidly. The loss of the misalignment detector will render the thermostat system useless.

The idea that both disturbance and misalignment detectors can be useful in control mechanisms is a very fruitful one in biology. Consider first the body's own temperature regulating mechanism as it operates in warm-blooded creatures. Which part of the body is most nearly maintained at a constant temperature? It is certainly not the skin for the skin temperature may fluctuate widely depending on the outside conditions. In fact the arterial blood has the most nearly constant temperature of all the body tissues and it therefore seems reasonable to suggest that it is the temperature of the arterial blood which the regulating systems attempt to keep constant. The relatively constant temperature of many other parts of the body merely indicates that they are well-supplied with arterial blood.

Misalignment detectors should therefore be located where they can monitor the temperature of arterial blood. Since the arterial blood supply to the nervous system is of over-riding importance, it might be expected that these detectors would be situated in the brain. This expectation has been found to be true and there is abundant evidence that the arterial temperature receptors are situated in the hypothalamus. Disturbance of hypothalamic function in humans because of vascular disease or by a tumour can produce severe derangement of temperature regulation. The body temperature may remain persistently high or persistently low.

The value of disturbance detectors

But as common experience indicates, temperature receptors are not only found in the brain. The skin is very obviously temperature sensitive and rapidly detects changes in the temperature of the environment. However, the skin receptors adapt quickly to new situations and in the steady state one is unaware that they are functioning. But the receptors do warn of temperature changes and they are ideal disturbance detectors. Many experiments have shown that they can function in this way. For example, if an animal is exposed to radiant heat, the blood flow to the skin is increased and sweating begins before any change can be detected in the arterial blood temperature. The information from the skin receptors enables the control system to anticipate a change in the blood temperature. Human beings and animals exposed to a hot sun will seek shade and thus reduce the heat stress long before the blood temperature has altered. In both cases the skin receptors act as disturbance detectors warning the control system that unless the rate of heat gain is reduced and the rate of heat loss is increased, the arterial blood temperature will rise. If the blood temperature rises because the heat stress is too great or if it falls because the measures set in motion to lower body temperature have been too energetic, this will be detected by the central hypothalamic receptors and the final fine control will operate. The control of arterial blood temperature would be less precise and the oscillations would be greater without the existence of disturbance detectors on the body surface.

What will happen if the two sets of receptors, central brain and superficial skin, provide conflicting information? If the central temperature receptors are behaving as true misalignment detectors while the skin ones are simply disturbance detectors, the information provided by the central ones should be dominant. Experiments of this type have been done. The arterial blood can be cooled either by placing a large volume of iced water in the stomach or by actually infusing cold salt solution into a vein. At the same time the skin can be kept very warm by keeping the subject of the experiment in a hot room. Under these conditions, even though the skin is warm, sweating falls to very low levels, skin blood flow is reduced and even shivering may occur. If the reverse experiment is done and the arterial blood is warmed while the skin is kept cold, sweating and skin blood flow both increase. Thus what actually happens is precisely what one would expect if the skin receptors were acting merely as disturbance detectors while the arterial blood receptors were acting as dominant misalignment detectors.

Another good example of the use of disturbance detectors can be seen in the control of the breathing during exercise. As mentioned earlier, once exercise is being done at a steady rate, the rate of ventilation seems to be determined by the rate of carbon dioxide production. As a result of the operation of arterial misalignment detectors for carbon dioxide, the rate of ventilation is so increased that the increased rate of carbon dioxide removal is just balanced by the increased rate of production. But when a person at rest suddenly begins to take exercise, it is some time before the increased muscular activity causes an increased outpouring of carbon dioxide into the venous blood. If the misalignment detectors for carbon dioxide were the only sources of information for the control of ventilation, there would be a finite time lag between the beginning of the exercise and the rise in the ventilation rate. What actually happens? Suppose we study the ventilation rate in someone sitting on a bicycle so mounted that it remains stationary when the pedals are turned. Suppose also that it is possible to apply a brake to the wheels so changing the resistance against which the pedals must be pushed. When a person who has been at rest suddenly begins pedalling, the ventilation rate rises sharply long before any change can be detected in the rate of carbon dioxide entry into the blood. This sudden increase is then followed by a further, slower rise until a steady rate of ventilation is reached which copes satisfactorily with a steady rate of exercise. If a series of separate tests is done in which the subject is asked to pedal against different resistances, it is found that the sudden initial increase is roughly the same whatever the resistance. However, the final plateau depends on the intensity of

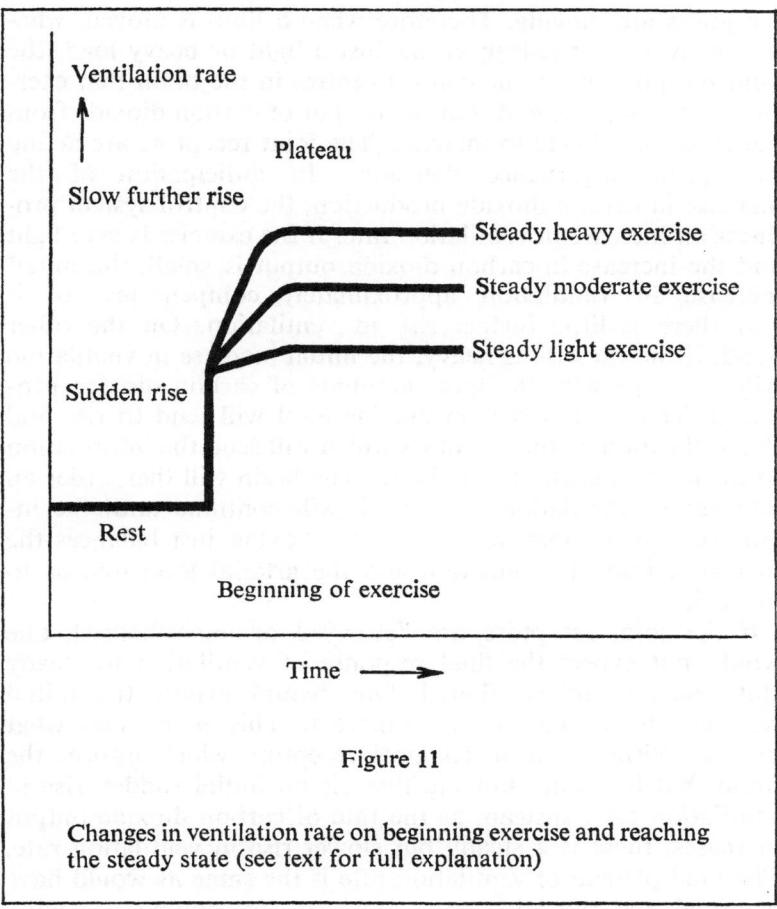

Figure 11

Changes in ventilation rate on beginning exercise and reaching the steady state (see text for full explanation)

the work being done, the harder the work, the greater is the second slower rise.

Experiments in animals have revealed that, as might be expected, the sharp initial rise does not depend on chemical changes in the blood. Instead it depends on the activation of mechanical receptors in the exercising limbs, particularly those in the joints which signal to the brain when and how rapidly

31

the joints are moving. Therefore when a limb is moved, whether actively or passively or against a light or heavy load, the joint receptors warn the control centres in the brain that exercise is taking place and that the output of carbon dioxide from the muscles is likely to increase. The joint receptors are acting as typical disturbance detectors. In anticipation of the increase in carbon dioxide production, the control system produces an increase in ventilation rate. If the exercise is very light and the increase in carbon dioxide output is small, the initial increase in ventilation approximately compensates for it and there is little further rise in ventilation. On the other hand, if the exercise is heavy, the initial increase in ventilation will not cope with the large amounts of carbon dioxide produced. The arterial carbon dioxide level will tend to rise and this will stimulate the receptors which will send the information to the control centre in the brain. The brain will then order an increase in ventilation rate which will continue until the increased rate of removal of carbon dioxide just balances the increased rate of production and the arterial level returns to normal.

If the joint receptors are destroyed or anaesthetised, one would not expect the final response of ventilation to steady state exercise to be altered. One would expect the initial response to change to be different. This is in fact what occurs. Without the mechanical receptors which inform the brain that limbs are moving there is no initial sudden rise in ventilation rate. Instead, as the rate of carbon dioxide output increases, there is a steady but slower rise in ventilation rate. The final plateau of ventilation rate is the same as would have occurred had the joint receptors been functioning normally. Therefore as would be expected from their function as disturbance detectors, the limb receptors influence the rate of response to change but not the magnitude of the final response.

The mechanisms controlling appetite and thirst provide further biological examples of situations where both disturbance and misalignment detectors are important. The sensation of thirst depends primarily on minute increases in the ionic

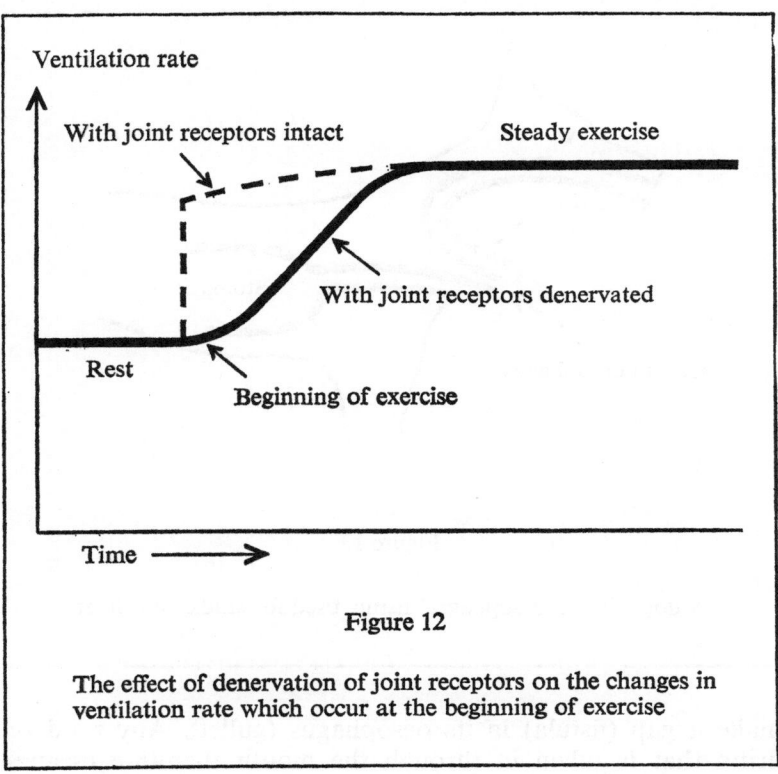

Figure 12

The effect of denervation of joint receptors on the changes in
ventilation rate which occur at the beginning of exercise

concentration of the blood which indicate that the body is being
depleted of water. The detection of these changes depends
again on receptors in the hypothalamus which monitor the
composition of the blood flowing through the brain. If the ionic
concentration rises above normal because of loss of water then
a sensation of intense thirst results. The situation can be produced artificially by injecting minute amounts of concentrated
salt solution into the carotid arteries which supply the
brain.

Suppose that the sensation of thirst is investigated in a dog
which has previously been subjected to an operation in order to

33

Principles of biological control

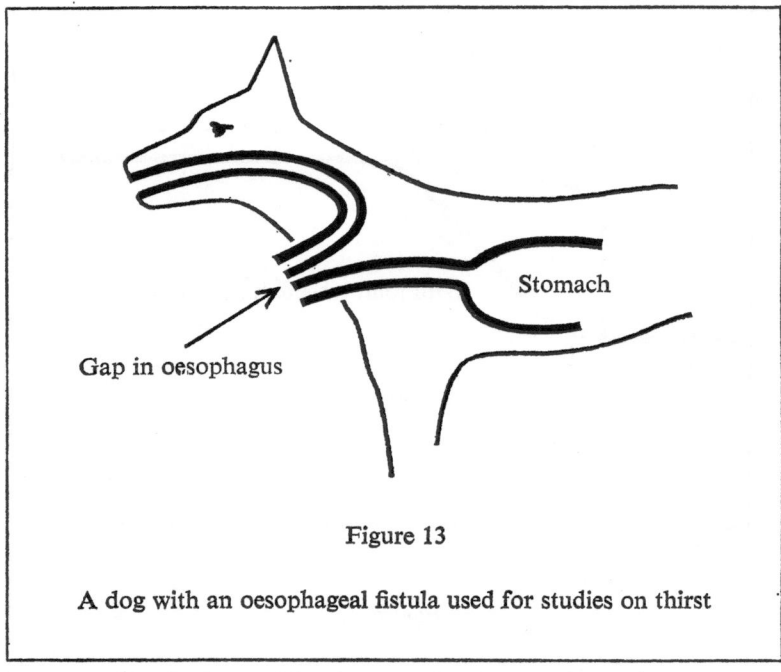

Figure 13

A dog with an oesophageal fistula used for studies on thirst

make a gap (fistula) in its oesophagus (gullet). Any food or drink that is taken in through the mouth therefore escapes from the gap in the oesophagus without entering the stomach. If the dog is deprived of water for a couple of days it will become very thirsty and blood sampling will reveal that the ionic concentration of the blood is above normal. What then happens if water is provided? The dog will drink voraciously and will continue drinking until it is exhausted because the water does not reach the stomach and intestines and therefore does not enter the body. On the other hand, suppose that in a thirsty dog a large volume of water is poured into the stomach before the dog is allowed to drink. When the animal is allowed access to water it will take just a few mouthfuls and then stop. If a blood sample is taken at this point it reveals that its sensation of thirst has vanished long before all the water in the stomach has been absorbed into the body and long before the chemical changes in the blood have been reversed to normal. Sensory receptors in the wall of the stomach which are stretched when the stomach is filled act as disturbance detectors informing the central control centre that the water deficit is likely to be made good. When after 30–60 minutes all the water has been absorbed, the more precise blood sampling receptors in the hypothalamus which act as misalignment detectors assess whether or not the deficit has been accurately replaced. If it has not the sensation of thirst may return.

The disturbance detectors are very important in the regulation of the body water content. Suppose that the misalignment detectors in the hypothalamus were the only receptors supplying information to the control system. Suppose that in order to abolish the sensation of thirst, drinking had to continue until the chemical changes in the blood were fully reversed to normal. After all ordinary degrees of dehydration, the amount of water required to replace the loss can be swallowed in a few minutes. But it may be thirty minutes or more before that water is absorbed from the gut and the chemical changes are corrected. If a human being or animal remained thirsty all that time, far more water would be swallowed than was actually required. By the time the chemical composition of the blood had returned to normal, large amounts of water would be left in the gut. The absorption of this water would dilute the blood and the kidney would have to work hard to excrete the excess in the form of urine.

Much the same considerations apply to appetite. The sensation of hunger almost certainly depends on subtle alterations in the carbohydrate and fat content of the blood which are by no means clearly understood as yet. Again the receptors which detect these changes seem to be in the hypothalamus. It is a matter of common experience that no matter how hungry one may be the sensation of hunger is greatly diminished by just a few mouthfuls. The sensation vanishes while most of the food is still in the gut being digested and long before any biochemical changes could have been reversed. Animal experiments have demonstrated that the sensation of hunger can be considerably reduced simply by stretching the stomach, even if the stretching is done by material which has no food value. Again the disturbance detectors are of obvious significance. If we ate until the biochemical changes in the blood were completely reversed, all meals would be orgies lasting several hours. When we had reached the stage of being no longer hungry, the gut would still be loaded with food and there would be no need to eat again for many hours more. We might therefore eat once per day or even once every several days. It is possible that appetite control in animals such as snakes may work in this way.

Chapter 5

The influence of the type of stress on the design of a control system

With some control mechanisms, outside stresses which tend to disturb the system always tend to push the system in one direction. With other control mechanisms, there may be several different types of outside stress, some tending to push the system in one direction and some tending to push it in the other. Control systems to cope with the second situation must be much more complex than those which can cope with the first. Concrete examples may help to demonstrate this.

Suppose that one built a submarine chamber beneath the Arctic ice cap. The chamber would be surrounded by water whose temperature remains at about 4°C all the year round. Suppose that one wanted to maintain the temperature inside the chamber at 20°C. The only source of heat supplied to the chamber would be the heating system actually installed in it. If as a result of the operation of the heating system the chamber became slightly too hot, the effect of the water outside would automatically cool it down as soon as the heating was turned down. A very simple control system could therefore maintain the temperature of the chamber constant all the year round.

In contrast, the problems of controlling the internal temperature of a house placed in the middle of a continent in one of the temperate regions of the world, say in Central Europe or the American Mid-West, are quite different. In winter the difficulties are similar to those experienced in the Arctic. All one needs is a heating system. If the heating system makes the house too hot, then all that is required is to turn the heating down. The cold outside will then lower the internal temperature in a satisfactory way. But this simple mechanism will be quite useless in the summer when the temperature outside may be much hotter than the temperature which is required inside. Simply turning off the heating will not then bring down the internal temperature to the required value. An active refrigeration system for cooling the air inside the house is required. Thus if the stress is always in one direction, one type of effector mechanism will suffice to achieve satisfactory control. If outside stresses can push the system either way from the desired set level, then at least two different effectors are required.

Some problems of biological control are similar to those of heating a chamber in the Arctic sea: the stress is always in one direction. For example, consider the control of the secretion of ACTH from the anterior pituitary. This depends only on the amount of CRF reaching the pituitary from the hypothalamus. ACTH output cannot be stimulated in any other way. If the pituitary is removed from its position at the base of the brain and transplanted to a quite different part of the body, it ceases to be exposed to the action of releasing factor in the normal way. The output of ACTH falls to zero and there are no external stresses which can increase it. Thus when the pituitary is in its normal position, by varying the output of releasing factor the output of ACTH can be varied over its full range. The one mechanism for controlling ACTH output will suffice and there is no need to invoke any other. Similar considerations apply to the control of the output of thyroid hormone by TSH. If TSH output is zero then the output of thyroid hormone is also zero. Again by varying the TSH output, the output of thyroid hormone can be varied over the full range required.

In contrast, there are several biological control mechanisms where one type of effector control is not sufficient. The problem of regulating blood glucose level is one such case. After a meal, when the food is being absorbed into the body from the gut, the blood glucose concentration tends to rise to very high levels. If the concentration is to be maintained within normal limits, it is essential to have a mechanism for bringing the level down. This is done very effectively by insulin. On the other hand, during exercise the muscles consume glucose extremely rapidly and there is a danger that the blood glucose level may fall. Since the brain depends almost entirely on glucose for its energy supply low glucose levels in the blood could clearly produce a dangerous situation with a risk of loss of consciousness. It is therefore not surprising that in order to counter this danger there are at least four mechanisms, all acting in different ways, which can raise the blood glucose level and maintain the supply to the brain. Growth hormone from the pituitary, cortisol from the adrenal cortex, glucagon from the pancreas and adrenaline from the adrenal medulla can all act to raise blood glucose. Thus because blood glucose may either tend to rise abnormally high or to fall abnormally low in different situations, there are active mechanisms for raising it and quite different ones for lowering it.

The temperature regulation of the body provides another instance. If the body temperature falls in a cold environment, heat production can be increased by exercise and by shivering and heat loss can be cut down by reducing the blood flow through the skin. If the environmental temperature is high and the body temperature rises, then heat production can be cut down by physical rest and heat loss can be increaed by active sweating and by an increase in the skin blood flow. The body must be able to resist disturbances of temperature in both directions and in each case different effector mechanisms are involved. The body possesses both active heating and active refrigeration systems.

Chapter 6

Systems with multiple detectors and multiple effectors

Biologists, working with organisms which contain by far the most complex computers known, often seem to take an unduly simple-minded view of the systems which they are studying. Their model of a control mechanism is all too often the household thermostat in its most basic form. This consists of one temperature measuring device, one control device, sensitive to changes in the thermometer reading, and one heating system which responds to the control device in an appropriate way.

Suppose you were in charge of the design of a temperature controlling system for a space capsule which was to be landed on Mars and which was going to be subjected to extremes of heat and cold. It would no doubt be very, very clear to you that the lives of the men inside the capsule would depend on the effective functioning of your system. If your system failed they would either freeze or fry. Would you be content therefore with installing in the capsule one thermometer, one controlling device and one heating and cooling system? I suggest that you would not. Your measuring system would consist of at least two thermometers and possibly more so that if one failed for any reason, the others could quickly take over and temperature regulation would continue to be effective. You might also install at least two controlling devices and two effector systems so that if one failed another could take over.

I venture to suggest that many of the body's controlling mechanisms, shaped by millions of years of fighting for survival in evolution are no less sophisticated. Most of the important

Systems with multiple detectors and effectors

factors in the body which must be precisely controlled are probably monitored by sense organs in several different sites. In most cases, too, there are probably several different mechanisms whereby a desired effector response can be brought about. The control of arterial blood pressure is an excellent illustration of what I mean. It is essential that under normal conditions the pressure of the blood in the arteries should be regulated within fairly narrow limits. If the pressure is too low, there may not be enough force to supply blood to the various organs: as a result the organs may die or be permanently damaged by the lack of blood. If the blood pressure is too high blood vessels in some organs may burst open and a great strain may be put on the heart. Because the control of blood pressure is so important one might expect that there would be several different receptors supplying information to the brain about it and several different effector mechanisms for controlling it.

This is indeed the case. There are pressure receptors in the walls of many different blood vessels. When the pressure inside the vessel rises, the walls are distended and the receptors are stretched. The higher the pressure the more nervous impulses are fired by the receptors and transmitted to the brain. The latter therefore receives a barrage of information about the pressure of the blood in many different arteries. The most important of these pressure receptors seem to be the ones in the carotid artery in the neck in the region of the artery known as the carotid sinus. They are in a good position to measure the pressure of the blood in the arteries which supply the brain. They send the information about pressure to the central control mechanism along what is known as the sinus nerve. What therefore happens if the sinus nerves on both sides of the neck are cut, thus stopping information about pressure reaching the brain via this pathway? Under normal circumstances, a fall in the number of nerve impulses travelling along the sinus nerve would indicate a fall in blood pressure. Initially in the experiment the brain is fooled. It does interpret the cutting of the nerve as a fall in blood pressure. In a vain effort to restore the discharge in the sinus nerves to normal levels, the

Principles of biological control

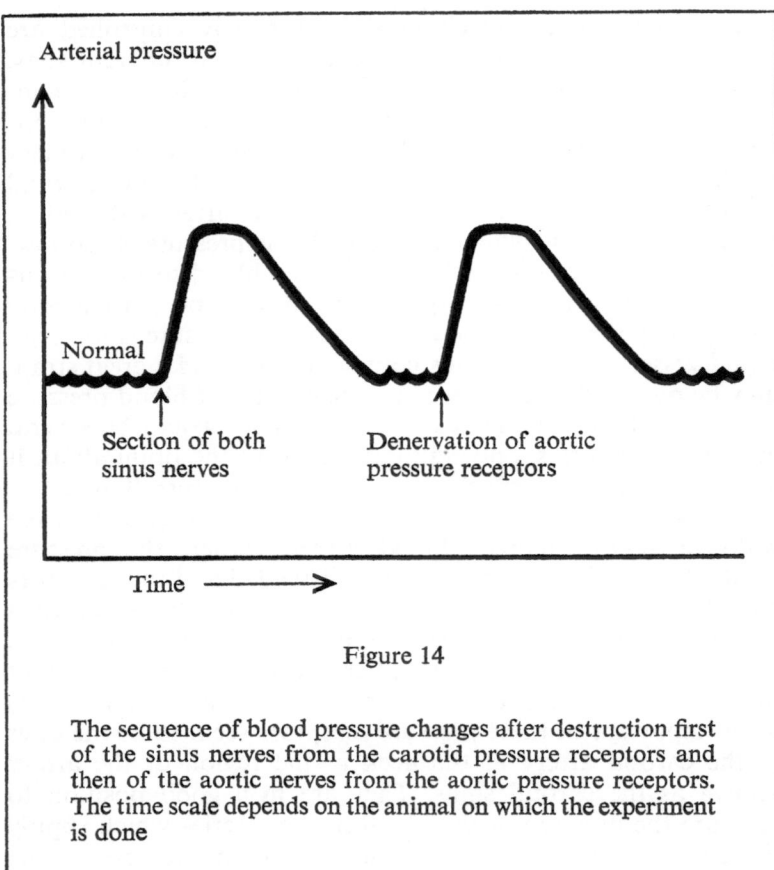

Figure 14

The sequence of blood pressure changes after destruction first of the sinus nerves from the carotid pressure receptors and then of the aortic nerves from the aortic pressure receptors. The time scale depends on the animal on which the experiment is done

brain sets in motion effector changes which raise the arterial pressure well above normal. The pressure remains high for a time but then gradually returns to normal levels even though the important sinus nerves have been destroyed. This return to normal arterial pressures is not difficult to understand.

There are many other arterial pressure receptors supplying information to the brain. These continually signal that the

42

arterial pressure is above normal. The control mechanism will rapidly be made aware of the discrepancy between the information from the sinus nerves and that from other pressure receptors.

Furthermore, assuming that the brain is a sophisticated computer, it will no doubt soon realise that there is no correlation between its attempts to raise arterial pressure by altering effector mechanisms and the activity in the sinus nerves. When the brain sets in motion mechanisms which raise arterial pressure, the sensory discharge in the pressure receptors normally rises accordingly. In this experiment nothing happens in the sinus nerves when the pressure is raised but the discharge from other receptors increases as usual.

The brain therefore ignores completely the lack of activity in the sinus nerves and relies entirely on information from elsewhere. The cycle is repeated if what appear to be the second most important pressure receptors, those in the aorta (the main artery which comes from the heart) are then denervated. Again the pressure rises initially but again it falls after a period as the normally less important pressure receptors in other arteries take over. It is important to note that if the receptors of secondary importance are destroyed while the sinus receptors are left intact, the blood pressure does not usually change. But that does not mean that the secondary receptors are of no significance. Like the secondary thermometers in the thermostat system of a spacecraft, their importance is revealed only when the primary receptors fail.

In controlling arterial pressure, the body is equally versatile on the effector side. The maintenance of a normal arterial pressure depends on the fact that the heart pumps out blood into a system of tubes which offers resistance to the flow of that blood. If the resistance remains constant, the more blood that is pumped out per minute the higher will be the pressure. The pressure therefore depends partly on the cardiac output, the amount of blood pumped out by the heart every minute. On the other hand, if the cardiac output remains constant but the resistance offered by the vessels becomes greater, the pressure will again rise. The reverse changes will produce a fall in arterial pressure. The resistance offered by the system of tubes can be altered because the walls of the small blood vessels are muscular. If the muscle in a vessel wall contracts, the diameter of that vessel becomes less and the resistance to blood flow increases. If the muscle relaxes, the resistance to flow will fall: if the cardiac output then remains constant, the arterial pressure will also fall.

And so the arterial pressure can be altered either by changing the resistance or by changing the cardiac output. But the mechanism is considerably more versatile even than that. The cardiac output itself can be altered in many different ways. To name but three of these, the output can be increased by an increase in the activity of the excitatory sympathetic nerves to the heart, by a decrease in the activity of the inhibitory vagal nerve fibres or by an increase in the concentration of the hormone adrenaline in the blood. Similarly the resistance offered by the blood vessels can also be altered in many different ways. Therefore if only one of the effector control mechanisms is damaged, any effect on the level of arterial pressure is likely to be only slight and temporary. The brain has at its disposal so many methods of altering both cardiac output and resistance that only if the majority of them cease to function is blood pressure likely to be permanently affected.

Thus in many biological situations only the naive would expect any permanent alteration if only one of several possible sources of information or only one of several possible effector mechanisms is destroyed. Despite this, biological history contains many examples of false reasoning based on the argument that a sensory receptor is insignificant in effect if its destruction is followed by virtually normal functioning of the body. That is rather like saying that if the temperature of a spacecraft remains steady after one of two available thermometers in the control system has been destroyed then the destroyed thermometer was functionless and unimportant. This is clearly nonsense because although the system still functions normally, one line of defence has gone and the spacecraft is less well placed to cope with further damage. The possession of many receptor and many effector mechanisms dealing with a single factor is a simple precaution of defence in depth forced upon successful organisms by many years of evolution.

With arterial pressure, although there are many receptors, theoretically the regulating system could function only with one since the pressure of the blood is essentially the same throughout the arterial tree. A similar thing is true of mechanisms which control the chemical composition of the blood. The concentrations in the blood of most substances are effectively identical throughout the vascular system. Only one receptor could do the job of monitoring the blood although in practice there may be several. However, some things which are kept constant by their very nature require the collection of information from many different sources. For example, in any one individual the volume of blood is kept remarkably constant. Yet there can obviously be no single simple way of measuring the volume of blood stored in such an extremely complicated system of tubes as the vascular system. The accurate system of blood volume must therefore depend on collecting information about the volume of blood in arteries, veins and in small vessels in many organs. Only by collecting information from many, many receptors and integrating that information in the brain can a reliable picture of the blood volume be compiled. If this is so it is unlikely that an experiment which investigates the effect on the control of blood volume of the destruction of just one or two likely receptors will have any positive result. All the other receptors involved will still be signalling "situation normal" and the brain will conclude that even if the cessation of information from the destroyed receptors means anything at all it cannot be very significant. Therefore if one denervates an organ which may be playing a role in the collection of information about blood volume and nothing happens then one is not entitled to conclude that that receptor is not involved in volume control.

Chapter 7

Alteration of the behaviour of control mechanisms

With most thermostats, even ones of very simple design, it is possible to alter the setting around which the control mechanism operates. The householder can decide whether he wishes the temperature of a room to be maintained at 10°C or 15°C or 20°C by turning a dial which alters the point at which the heating and cooling systems turn on and off. Many of the body's control mechanisms appear to have similar devices which may either alter the behaviour of a sensory receptor or without altering the behaviour of the receptor may alter the way in which the central control mechanism responds to the information provided.

A mechanism which clearly illustrates the two ways in which a control system can be altered is that of the emptying of the large bowel (defaecation). The wall of the large bowel contains sensory receptors which are sensitive to stretch. The receptors are arranged so that they are in series with muscle fibres in the bowel wall. There are therefore two ways in which the sense organs can be stretched.

1. By an increase in the volume of the contents of the bowel.
2. By contraction of the muscles in the wall of the bowel.

When the receptors are stretched, the information is sent back to a control centre in the spinal cord. When the receptor discharge reaches a critical level the control centre orders emptying of the bowel. In infants and in paraplegics (patients who have had their spinal cord cut across), the mechanism operates

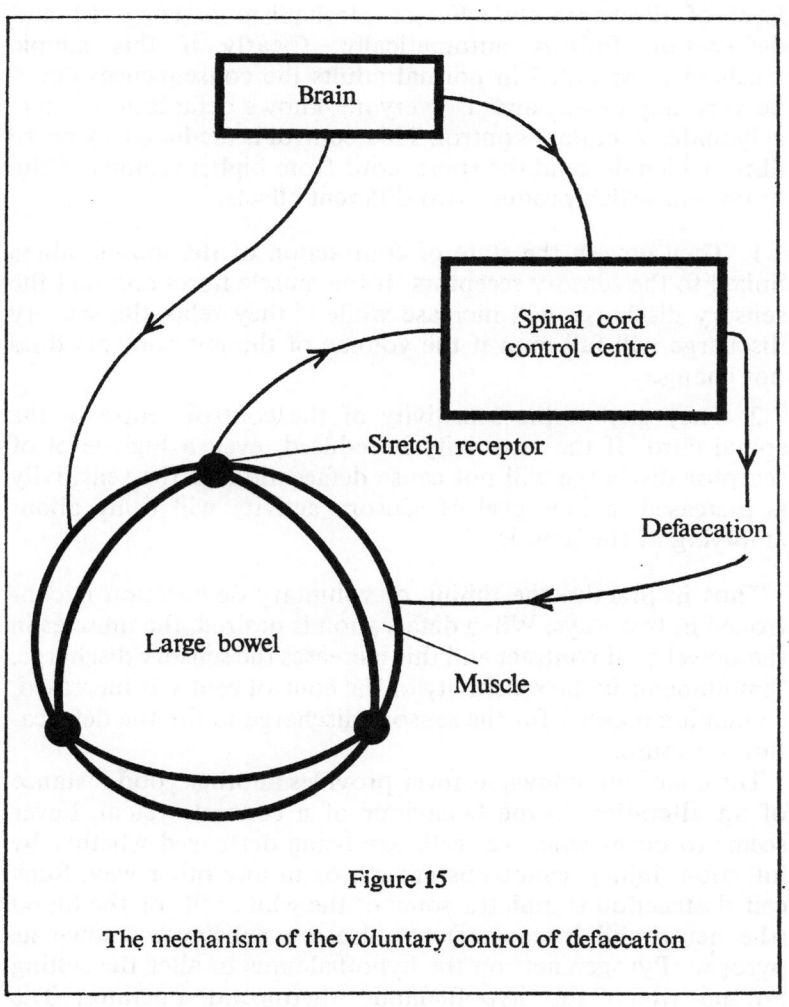

Figure 15

The mechanism of the voluntary control of defaecation

in this simple way. As the large bowel becomes loaded with faeces the receptors are stretched more and more. At a certain level of discharge the effector mechanism is triggered and defaecation follows automatically. Clearly if this simple mechanism operated in normal adults the consequences could be very unpleasant and as everyone knows defaecation is largely under voluntary control. This control is mediated by nerve fibres which descend the spinal cord from higher regions of the brain and which produce two different effects.

1. They govern the state of contraction of the muscle fibres linked to the sensory receptors. If the muscle fibres contract the sensory discharge will increase while if they relax the sensory discharge will fall even if the volume of the gut contents does not change.

2. They govern the sensitivity of the control centre in the spinal cord. If the sensitivity is reduced, even a high level of receptor discharge will not cause defaecation. If the sensitivity is increased, a low level of sensory activity will bring about emptying of the bowel.

Thus in practice the timing of voluntary defaecation is controlled in two ways. When defaecation is desired, the muscles in the bowel wall contract and this increases the sensory discharge. Simultaneously the sensitivity of the control centre is increased, so making it easier for the sensory discharge to fire the defaecation response.

The condition known as fever provides another good instance of an alteration in the behaviour of a control system. Fever seems to occur whenever cells are being destroyed whether by infection, injury, cancerous growth or in any other way. Such cell destruction stimulates some of the white cells of the blood (the neutrophil leucocytes) to release a substance known as pyrogen. Pyrogen acts on the hypothalamus to alter the setting around which the hypothalamic thermostat operates. The function of the response is not clear and as yet there is little evidence that it helps to protect the body against disease.

Alteration of behaviour of control mechanisms

Nevertheless it does occur and its mode of operation is well known.

The arterial blood temperature is normally regulated around the level of 37°C. If it rises above this, the skin blood flow increases and sweating occurs in order to bring it back to normal. If the temperature falls below 37°C, heat production may be increased by shivering and heat loss reduced by cutting down skin blood flow until the temperature returns again to normal.

What then happens at the beginning of fever? Even though the temperature is normal, heat production is increased by shivering and heat loss is reduced by cutting down the skin blood flow. The body temperature therefore rises until it reaches a new equilibrium level, say 39°C. If then the body temperature is artificially reduced to 38°C by cold sponging or by the infusion of cold saline, shivering sets in and the temperature soon rises again. Yet in a normal individual, a temperature of 38°C would produce quite the opposite reactions, namely sweating and increased skin blood flow. The pyrogen has clearly shifted the setting of the thermostat. When the pyrogen level falls at the end of fever, the setting reverts to 37°C and the temperature is brought back to normal by excess sweating and increased skin blood flow.

Yet another exmple may be taken from the field of endocrine physiology. ACTH is released from the anterior pituitary under the influence of its releasing factor, CRF. The amount of CRF produced by the hypothalamus depends on the amount of cortisol in the circulating blood. If the cortisol concentration rises above a certain critical level, X, the amount of releasing factor put out falls. If the cortisol level falls below X, the CRF output rises. The changes in CRF, acting via ACTH, ultimately produce corresponding changes in the rate of the synthesis of cortisol by the adrenal cortex. Therefore the level of cortisol in the blood remains approximately constant. But the setting of the cortisol-CRF link can be altered by several other factors. One of these is any form of stress, whether physical or psychological, imposed on the individual. Information about the

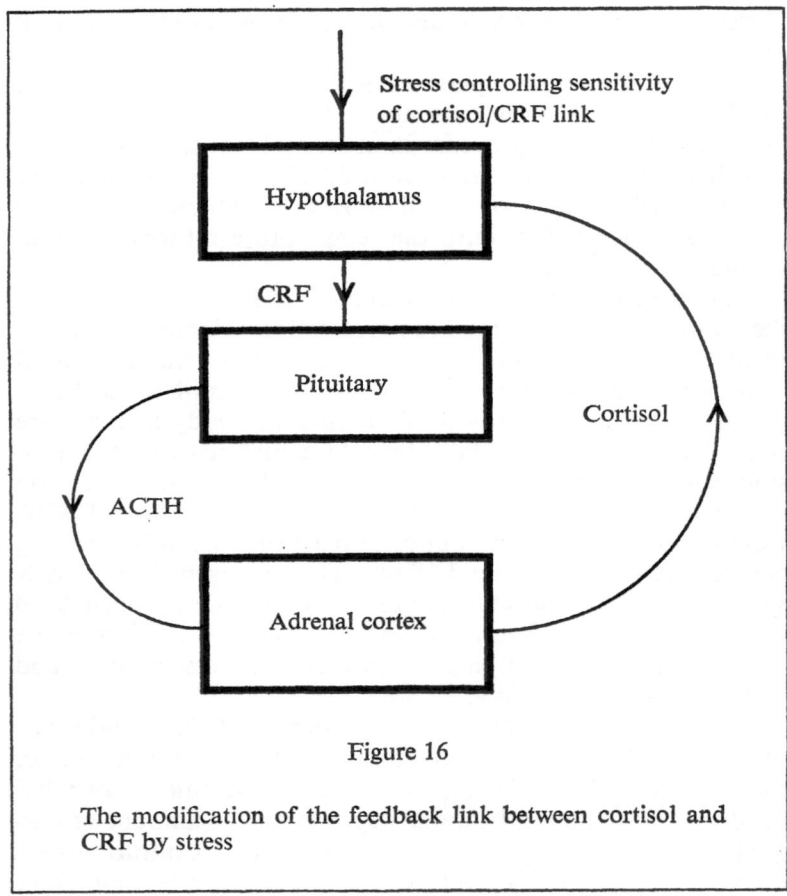

Figure 16

The modification of the feedback link between cortisol and CRF by stress

stress is conveyed to the hypothalamus where it leads to a reduction in the sensitivity of the CRF response to cortisol. Even though the concentration of cortisol in the blood may be X, this is now insufficient to control the output of CRF. The rate of CRF release is therefore increased, ACTH and hence cortisol outputs rise, and eventually at a new level of blood cortisol (X + Y), the output of CRF becomes stabilised. In the new situation if the cortisol level rises above (X + Y) the output of CRF decreases: if the level falls below (X + Y) the output of CRF increases. At the end of the period of stress, the sensitivity of the hypothalamic mechanism returns to its old level and the concentration of blood cortisol falls back to X.

An instance which has not been so well established as the others so far discussed is that of the control of the sensitivity of the arterial pressure receptors. All of these receptors seem to be in arterial walls. They can all be influenced by the state of contraction of the muscle in the wall in the same way as can the pressure receptors in the bowel which control defaecation. Suppose that the central control mechanism in the brain requires that under normal conditions the rate of sensory receptor discharge should be X. It is clear that this discharge may be influenced by three factors:

1. The pressure of blood within the vessel.
2. The state of contraction of the muscle fibres within the arterial wall.
3. The stiffness of the arterial wall. The stiffer it is the greater will be the pressure required to produce a given rate of receptor discharge.

Suppose for the moment that the stiffness remains constant, and simply consider the blood pressure and the degree of muscle contraction. Suppose that the component of receptor discharge attributable to the blood pressure is A, while that attributable to muscular contraction is B. Under normal circumstances A + B must equal X. What will then happen to the arterial pressure if the muscle tension increases? The receptors will be stretched and B will rise: the total receptor discharge will therefore rise above X. Receptor discharge can be brought back to X only if A, the component of the discharge attributable to the arterial blood pressure, falls. And this is just what happens. If adrenaline (epinephrine), which stimulates muscle to contract, is put on the wall of the carotid artery, the discharge of the pressure receptors there rises, even though initially the blood pressure is normal. The rate of discharge can be

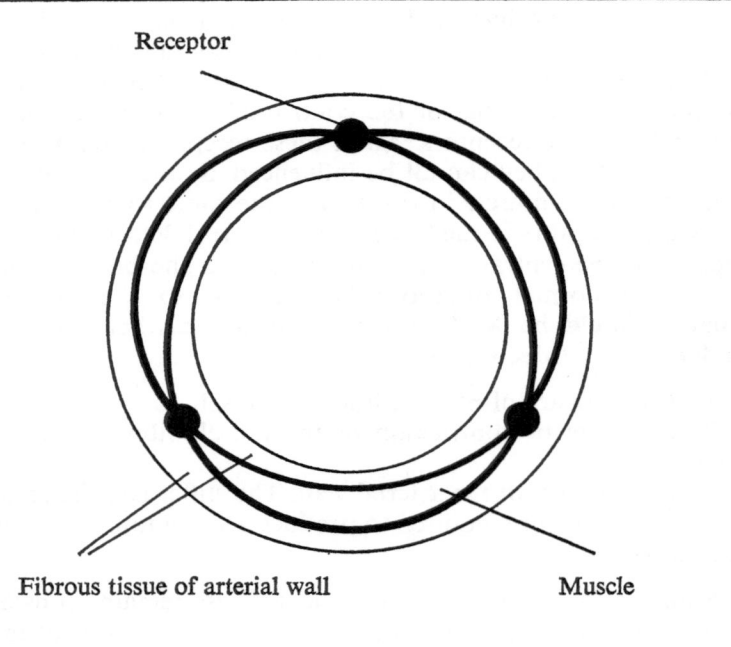

Receptor

Fibrous tissue of arterial wall   Muscle

Figure 17

Schematic outline of the factors which may influence the
function of the arterial blood pressure receptors. The receptors
may be stretched either by a rise of the blood pressure inside
the vessel or by contraction of the muscle fibres in the wall.
If the fibrous tissue of the vessel wall becomes stiffer, a higher
blood pressure will be required to produce the same degree of
receptor stretch.

reduced to its normal level only if the arterial blood pressure falls and this is what actually happens. The central control so alters the behaviour of the effectors that the blood pressure falls until it is stabilised when the receptor activity returns to its original level. If nitrites, which relax muscle, are put on the arterial wall, precisely the opposite happens. The arterial pressure rises in order to compensate for the fall in receptor discharge produced by the muscle relaxation.

The significance of this phenomenon in the control of arterial pressure is uncertain. Most research workers deny its importance. It seems to me, however, that circulating hormones, among other things might well alter the state of contraction of the muscle and therefore alter blood pressure. But this is very much a personal view and is by no means generally accepted.

Chapter 8

Implications for research

A great deal of research in biology and medicine is concerned with the investigation of the behaviour of control systems. A knowledge of the simple principles of how biological control systems operate as outlined in this short book may be very helpful in planning an attack on a problem. When considering any control system there are several questions which should be asked.

1. What is the factor which remains constant when the organism is subjected to changing conditions? The factor which remains constant in value is likely to be the one which is being precisely controlled by the body. For example, when the body is exposed to different environments, the skin temperature may change remarkably but the arterial blood temperature remains nearly constant. It is therefore the arterial blood temperature which is being controlled. Or when an animal exercises, its rate of breathing may change considerably but the arterial carbon dioxide level remains virtually constant. It therefore seems likely that the rate of breathing is precisely regulated so that the arterial carbon dioxide level does remain steady.

2. Where are the receptors which monitor the state of the factor which is being controlled? These are the misalignment detectors. It is essential to remember that body control mechanisms are often highly sophisticated and that more than one receptor may be supplying information. In this case, if the

function of one receptor is destroyed it may have little apparent effect on the operation of the mechanism. But that does not mean that the receptor which has been inactivated is not an important part of the regulating system.

3. Are there any disturbance detectors which collect information, not about the factor which is being precisely regulated but about changes in the environment, whether external or internal, which may alter the state of the regulated factor? The skin temperature receptors, for instance, do not monitor the temperature of the arterial blood. But they do warn the central controlling mechanism of changes in skin temperature which are likely sooner or later to alter the arterial blood temperature. This information enables the control centre to anticipate the changes and to take evading action. Similarly, the joint receptors although they provide no direct information about the blood carbon dioxide level, do warn the respiratory control centre that movement is occurring and that the rate of carbon dioxide production is likely to be increased. Disturbance detectors have no effect in steady state situations. It is the response to change which they influence and the speed of the response is reduced if the disturbance detectors cease to function. Oscillations around the set level will therefore be greater than normal.

4. Where is the control centre which collects the information and alters the behaviour of the effectors correspondingly? In most cases the information is collected by nerves and sent to the central nervous system. The control centre is usually situated in the brain or spinal cord. In some cases, however, and this is more likely when hormones are involved, the control mechanism may be somewhere else. The parathyroid glands produce hormones which control the level of blood calcium. The output of these hormones is directly determined by the concentration of calcium in the blood reaching the glands. As far as is known, the nervous system is in no way involved and therefore the control must be biochemical and act within the gland itself.

5. What effector mechanisms are available to alter the level of the factor which is being controlled? Again it is as well to

55

remember that the body is highly sophisticated and that it is common for a factor to be controllable in several different ways, thus giving defence in depth. If one of the effector mechanisms is destroyed there may be others available to take over. It is often said that in formulating scientific hypotheses one should start with the simplest possible explanation of a phenomenon and test whether that is adequate. If it is, then more complex explanations are not required. This is perfectly valid. Unfortunately many research workers do not seem to understand it properly. They interpret it as meaning that simple explanations are always likely to be more correct than complex ones. This is by no means always true. The history of biology is littered with sad stories which illustrate this. For example, it is not uncommon for one group of investigators to say that it is the behaviour of receptor A which governs the output of hormone X. Another group says that this is nonsense and that all the evidence indicates that receptor B is the important one. A slanging match develops with each side asserting that its own simple explanation is completely right while the other explanation is completely wrong. Only after years of wasted effort does a still small voice of sanity intervene and point out that the system is complex and sophisticated and that information from both A and B receptors is used in controlling the output of hormone X.

Chapter 9

Application of control theory to a particular research problem—high arterial pressure

I wish to conclude this book by discussing the problem of the regulation of arterial pressure in the light of a knowledge of the principles on which control mechanisms work. High arterial pressure is one of the most important unsolved problems in medicine and in the vast majority of cases its cause is completely unknown. Many individuals, particularly those in older age groups, have an arterial pressure which is well above normal. This high pressure, or hypertension as it is called, has many deleterious effects. It increases the strain on the heart and may eventually cause heart failure. It damages the small blood vessels, particularly those in the brain, the eye and the kidney. Damage to the brain vessels may cause a stroke, damage to the eye may cause blindness, damage to the kidney may cause renal failure. Hypertension is common and is responsible for a large part of the suffering and death in the modern world.

The aim of the investigation of hypertension is to discover in each case the underlying cause which makes the blood pressure rise above normal levels. If the cause can be discovered, then treatment can be directed at it and is likely to be more rational and successful than it is at present. But unfortunately research in hypertension seems to have reached something of an impasse. Many apparently promising lines of investigation have proved fruitless and in the great majority of cases the reason for the rise in pressure is unknown. Most frequently, no abnormality of any other organ is associated with the pressure increase: the arterial pressure simply seems to rise for no reason at all. This condition is called essential hypertension and it is a complete mystery. In some cases, kidney disease or the partial blockage of a renal artery is followed by the development of high arterial pressure. The damage to the kidney has clearly in some way caused the high pressure but the factors involved are unknown. A few years ago the cause of this type of hypertension seemed clear but it has now been demonstrated that the proposed explanation is invalid (see appendix for a further discussion of this). Therefore we do not know why kidney disease should upset the pressure regulating mechanism. Again, hypertension may follow the growth of a tumour of the adrenal cortex which pours out large amounts of such hormones as cortisol or aldosterone. Obviously the hormones in some way cause the pressure rise, but the precise sequence of events is mysterious. In only one rare disease is the cause of the high blood pressure clear and that is the condition known as phaeochromocytoma. This is a tumour of the adrenal medulla or of similar tissue which may secrete enormous quantities of noradrenaline and adrenaline (norepinephrine and epinephrine). These hormones are particularly effective in raising arterial pressure because they act on both the factors which govern that pressure, the cardiac output and the resistance. The heart is stimulated to beat both faster and more vigorously. Many of the resistance vessels are narrowed and so the resistance against which the blood must be pumped out increases. The regulating mechanisms cannot cope with such large alterations in the behaviour of effector organs and so the arterial pressure rises. But this is the only example where we genuinely know the precise cause of the hypertension. And it is very rare.

In all other types of hypertension the mechanism of the pressure rise is unknown. Even more puzzling, in all types with the exception of phaeochromocytoma, the blood flow through the organs is normal. The cardiac output is also normal and the high pressure seems to be due to a uniform increase in resistance. The higher pressure compensates for the higher resistance and so the flow is normal. In contrast, in phaeochromocytoma, the blood flow through the skin, kidneys and gut vessels is exceptionally low in comparison to the flow through other organs. This is because the effects of adrenaline and noradrenaline on the vessels in these organs are particularly potent.

Most research in hypertension has been directed at the effector side of the pressure control mechanism. Most workers seem to feel that the initial event which first pushes up the pressure is an abnormally functioning effector which acts by raising either the cardiac output or the peripheral resistance. For the following reasons I should like to suggest that it is inherently unlikely that the initial disturbance in function should be on the effector side:

1. At least in the early stages, it is unlikely that more than one of the many regulating mechanisms for the effector control of arterial pressure will go wrong. If one does go wrong, and the pressure rises as a result, this will be detected by the pressure receptors and the information will be sent to the control centre in the brain. The control centre will have at its disposal many other normal effectors operating in many different ways. It will therefore be able to compensate for the abnormally functioning effector and will return blood pressure to normal.

2. The truth of the first point is emphasised by the fact that it is impossible to produce sustained hypertension by a continuous infusion of adrenaline at concentrations which are at all safe. This seems to be true of both man and animals. When the infusion into a vein is started the pressure rises to high levels which is not surprising since as mentioned earlier, adrenaline acts both on the heart and on the resistance vessels. However, within a short time, even though the intravenous infusion is continued, the arterial pressure falls to normal. The control mechanism must have found a way of compensating by altering the behaviour of other effector mechanisms. The existence of these other effector mechanisms is emphasised by the fact that when the adrenaline infusion is suddenly stopped, they can act

unopposed and the blood pressure falls to very low levels before gradually returning to normal. In phaeochromocytoma the hypertension must be produced by overwhelming amounts of adrenaline and noradrenaline secreted over many years. In the real disease, the existence of effector mechanisms opposing the action of the hormones is demonstrated by the fact that immediately the tumour is removed there is often a profound and dangerous fall in arterial pressure.

3. There seem to be many different causes of hypertension (e.g. renal disease, tumours producing cortisol, tumours producing aldosterone and so on). Although not impossible, it seems unlikely that if all these acted by interfering with effector function, they should all act on the same effector. Some might be expected to increase the heart rate, some the force with which the heart beats, some the resistance in some organs, some the resistance in other organs and so on. One would not expect the cardiac output and the distribution of blood flow to be normal in every case. Since this happens it means that all but one type must produce the same defect in effector function. It is significant that in phaeochromocytoma, the only type of hypertension which is certainly caused by an effector defect, the pattern of blood flow through the various organs is clearly abnormal.

4. The fact that the functioning of the effectors seems similar in all types of hypertension apart from phaeochromocytoma could be accounted for if the defects were in the receptors or in the central control mechanism. Suppose that the receptors fired fewer nerve impulses at a normal arterial pressure. In order to raise the sensory information to its usual level, the control centre would raise arterial pressure. Or suppose that the central mechanism became less sensitive and that it "required" a higher level of receptor discharge than normal. Again the arterial pressure would be raised. In both cases the control mechanism might use similar effector mechanisms. Thus several different defects on the sensory side or in the central control system could produce the same pattern of increased effector activity. It

is perhaps time that a more serious search was made on the receptor side for the differences between the various types of hypertension.

It is easy to see how many different factors could alter the working of the sensory side. Although the pressure receptors are numerous, they are unlike the effectors in that they all appear to work on the same principle. They are all stretch receptors embedded in a fibrous arterial wall, and they can all be influenced by the state of contraction of muscle fibres in the wall. If the fibrous tissue of the arterial wall becomes stiff for any reason, then all arteries and all receptors are likely to be similarly affected. Higher pressure will be required to stretch the stiffer wall to a normal degree and therefore hypertension will occur. The walls of arteries seem to become stiffer in old age, and this could perhaps account for the occurrence of essential hypertension whose frequency increases with increasing age. On the other hand, in children in whom the arterial wall is very soft and easily stretched, then a low arterial pressure will produce a normal receptor discharge. As the child grows up and fibrous tissue of the wall becomes stiffer, then higher pressures will be required to maintain the discharge at normal levels.

Equally, if some factor such as a hormone altered the state of contraction of the muscle in arterial walls, again all the pressure receptors would be similarly affected. If the muscle relaxed, then a higher pressure would be required to stretch the receptors normally, while if the muscle contracted a lower pressure would suffice.

Finally, if the behaviour of the central control mechanism were to be altered in some way, again a higher pressure might be required. This is a view which has been ably championed by Dickinson.

Whatever is the truth, a knowledge of the principles on which control systems work certainly suggests that a defect on the sensory side or in the control centre is a more likely cause of hypertension than a defect on the effector side. A defect on the effector side cannot explain why the circulatory pattern seems to be the same in almost all forms of hypertension. Nor can it explain why the control system does not employ other normally functioning effectors to bring the pressure back to normal. In contrast, many different defects on the sensory side or in the control centre might be compensated for by the same changes in effector function. Furthermore, since the control mechanism is entirely dependent on sensory information there is no way in which it can counteract defects on the sensory side or in the control centre itself. It is therefore a pity that more effort is not being directed to research on this aspect of blood pressure regulation.

Further reading

Elementary Books on Physiology
Introduction to Human Physiology, J. H. Green, Oxford Medical Publications, 2nd edition, 1968.
The Human Organism, D. F. Horrobin, Basic Books, New York, 1966.

Textbooks of Physiology
General Physiology, H. Davson, Churchill, London, 3rd ed. 1964.
Medical Physiology and Biochemistry, D. F. Horrobin, Edward Arnold, London, Williams & Wilkins, Baltimore, 1968.
Physiology, edited E. E. Selkurt, Little Brown, Boston, Churchill, London, 2nd ed. 1966.
Textbook of Medical Physiology, A. C. Guyton, Saunders, 3rd ed. 1968.
Review of Medical Physiology, W. F. Ganong, Lange, California, Blackwell, Oxford, 4th ed. 1969.

Temperature Regulation
"Adaptations to Cold", L. Irving, *Sc. Amer.*, Jan. 1966.
"Adaptation to Environment", *American Physiological Society Handbook of Physiology*, Section 4, 1964.
"Temperature Regulation", W. I. Cranston, *Brit. Med. J. 2*, 69, 1966.
"The Camel", K. Schmidt-Nielsen, *Sc. Amer.*, Dec. 1959.
"The Human Thermostat", T. H. Benzinger, *Sc. Amer.*, Jan. 1961.

Control of Breathing
"Physiology of Exercise", C. B. Chapman and J. H. Mitchell, *Sc. Amer.*, May 1965.
Physiology of Respiration, J. H. Comroe, Year Book Medical Publishers, Chicago, 1965.
"Respiration", *American Physiological Society Handbook of Physiology*, Section 3, 2 vols. 1964 and 1965.
Respiration, P. Dejours, Oxford University Press, 1966.

Nerve Impulse
"Nerve Impulses in Squid Axons", R. D. Keynes, *Sc. Amer.*, Dec. 1958.
Nerve, Muscle and Synapse, B. Katz, McGraw-Hill, New York and Maidenhead, 1966.
The Conduction of the Nervous Impulse, A. L. Hodgkin, Liverpool University Press, 1964.
"The Nerve Axon", P. F. Baker, *Sc. Amer.*, Mar. 1966.

Principles of biological control

Pituitary, Endocrine Glands and Ovulation

Brain-Thyroid Relationships, Ciba Foundation Study Group 18, Churchill, London, 1964.

"Hypothalamic Control of ACTH Release", G. Sayer, *Physiologist*, *4*, 56, 1961.

Hypothalamic Factors Releasing Pituitary Hormones, R. Guillemin, Recent Progr. Horm. Res. *20*, 1964.

"Regulation of Synthesis and Release of ACTH", J. Vernikos-Danellis, *Vitamins & Hormones*, *23*, 1965.

"The Female Sex Cycle", D. F. Horrobin, *J. Theoret, Biol.* 22, 80, 1968.

The Pituitary Gland, ed. G. W. Harris and B. T. Donovan, 4 vols, Butterworth, London, 1966.

Blood Pressure Regulation

Circulation, American Physiological Society Handbook of Physiology, 3 vols, 1962, 1963 and 1965.

High Blood Pressure, G. W. Pickering, Churchill, London, 2nd ed. 1968.

Neurogenic Hypertension, C. J. Dickinson, Blackwell Scientific Publications, Oxford, 1965.

Physiology and Biophysics of the Circulation, A. C. Burton, Year Book Medical Publishers, Chicago, 1965.

Reflexogenic Areas of the Cardiovascular System, C. Heymans and E. Neil, Churchill, London, 1958.

Renal Hypertension, ed. I. H. Page and J. W. McCubbin, Year Book Medical Publishers, Chicago, 1968.

"Some Effects of Long-term Progesterone Treatment in Rabbits and their Relevance to Pre-eclampsia", D. F. Horrobin, *Lancet*, *1*, 170, 1968.

"Theory of Hypertension", D. F. Horrobin, *Lancet 1*, 574, 1966.

Appendix

Renal hypertension

In the mid 1930's Goldblatt demonstrated that arterial pressure could be chronically raised by putting clamps on the renal arteries to restrict the flow of blood to the kidneys. This technique offered an ideal model for the study of the hypertension known to be associated with renal disease. Since then research on this topic has been intensive. A few years ago it seemed that the answer to the problem of renal hypertension was at hand. Clamping the renal arteries or damaging the kidneys in a number of different ways, stimulated the kidneys to secrete a substance called renin. This is an enzyme which can act on a protein in the blood to split off a small fragment known as angiotensin. In turn, angiotensin can stimulate the adrenal cortex to increase its output of the hormone aldosterone. Angiotensin turned out to be a very powerful constrictor of small blood vessels. It was capable of raising arterial blood pressure to very high levels by increasing the resistance against which the heart had to work. There seemed little doubt that renal hypertension was caused by an excess of angiotensin in the circulating blood.

Sadly, the whole field has again been thrown into confusion by actual measurements of the blood levels of renin and angiotensin in normal animals and humans and in those with renal hypertension. As yet the measurements of renin and angiotensin are not very accurate but nevertheless the implication of the work is clear. When clamps are put on the renal arteries or when the kidneys are damaged in certain ways, the blood pressure rises quickly as does the output of renin and angiotensin. In this early phase the angiotensin undoubtedly causes the high pressure. But unfortunately within a few days the blood levels of renin and angiotensin begin to fall. Yet despite this the blood pressure remains very high. In chronic renal hypertension, the blood levels of renin, angiotensin and aldosterone are near normal. It is possible that they may be slightly raised but the methods of measurement are not yet precise enough to be able to make a certain judgment on this point. What is certain is that the concentration of angiotensin is not high enough to account for the high arterial pressure on the basis of a direct action on the small vessels and so the mechanism of renal hypertension remains unknown.

As is usual, most attention has been directed to possible disturbances of effector function and little notice has been taken of the receptor side. It seems to me that the most likely explanation of the chronic hypertension is that the relatively low levels of renin, angiotensin, aldosterone, or of some other substance produced by the kidneys, alter the behaviour of the arterial wall receptors. If the receptors were made less sensitive, then a higher arterial blood pressure would be required to make them discharge in the normal way. In order to return the receptor discharge to normal, the central control mechanism would bring about the required increase in pressure. There are two crucial pieces of evidence in favour of this concept.

First of all, it is possible to record the behaviour of the sinus nerve fibres in normal animals and in ones with renal hypertension. If the sensitivity of the pressure receptors were normal, one would expect them to be much more active in the hypertensive animals, signalling furiously that the arterial pressure was well above normal. But this is not the case at all. Receptor activity is similar in the normal and in the hypertensive animals. The receptor discharge in the hypertensive animals is normal, even though the arterial blood pressure is well above normal. This can mean only one thing: in the animals with renal hypertension the receptors must be much less sensitive than usual. This change is usually dismissed as merely being a consequence of the high pressure. If this is so it is very odd that the receptor discharge should be so near normal, since if the loss in sensitivity is a consequence, there is no obvious reason why it should not be either lower or higher than normal. I submit that the change in sensitivity is much more likely to be the *cause* of the hypertension. I suggest that a change in receptor sensitivity brought about either by a change in the stiffness of the arterial wall fibrous tissue or by a change in the behaviour of the muscle in the arterial wall is the underlying mechanism behind chronic renal hypertension. The normality of the receptor discharge is a powerful argument in support of the view that the change in receptor behaviour is the cause of the hypertension.

Secondly, in an animal with chronic renal hypertension, destruction of the sympathetic nervous system brings about a profound fall in the blood pressure. Initially it seems as though the cause of the high pressure is therefore excessive activity of these sympathetic nerves. But within a short time, the arterial blood pressure rises again to its original level. Clearly other effector mechanisms have taken over. This is precisely the sequence of events one would expect if the defect in pressure regulation were on the sensory side. If the renal damage reduced in some way the sensitivity of the arterial pressure receptors, then a normal pressure would no longer produce a normal sensory discharge. The control centre in the brain would raise the pressure in order to return the sensory discharge to normal. Initially it might well use the sympathetic system as its main effector agent. If the sympathetic system were then destroyed, blood pressure would fall and with it the discharge of the sensory receptors. The control centre would then be expected to respond by bringing other effectors into play. The pressure would again rise until the receptor discharge became normal.

These logical arguments do not prove that the defect in the pressure regulating system is on the sensory side. But they do suggest that the idea is worth more consideration than has hitherto been given to it.

Index

ACTH (adrenocorticotrophic hormone), 6, 8, 18, 38, 49–51
ADH (anti-diuretic hormone, vasopressin), 6
Adrenal cortex, 2, 6, 18, 39, 49–51, 58
Adrenaline (epinephrine), 39, 44, 51, 58, 59, 60
Adrenal medulla, 39, 58
Adrenocorticotrophic hormone (ACTH), 6, 8, 18, 38, 49–51
Aldosterone, 58, 60
American Mid-West, 37
Angiotensin, 65 ff
Anti-diuretic hormone (ADH, vasopressin), 6
Aorta, 43
Appetite, 32 ff
Arctic, 37
Arterial pressure, 4, 15, 41 ff, 51 ff, 57 ff, 65 ff
Arteries, 4, 41, 45, 51 ff, 57 ff

Bicarbonate, 2
Blood, 4 ff, 13, 15, 18, 29, 30, 33, 38, 43 ff
  pressure, 4, 15, 41 ff, 51 ff, 57 ff, 65 ff
  volume, 45
Bowel, large, 46 ff
Brain, 4, 5, 6, 18, 28, 29, 32, 33, 39, 41, 43, 45, 47, 55, 57, 67
Breasts, 6
Breathing (ventilation), 4, 13, 15, 16, 18, 30, 54

Calcium, 2, 8, 55
Capillaries, 7, 8, 15
Carbohydrate, 1, 35
Carbon dioxide, 1, 4, 13, 15, 18, 26, 30, 54, 55

Carotid arteries, 33, 41, 51, 52
  sinus, 41 ff, 51 ff, 66, 67
Cells, 1 ff
  white, 48, 49
Central Europe, 37
Chemical composition, 1 ff, 35
Circulatory system, 4
Control systems, 9 ff, 37 ff, 53 ff
Cortex, adrenal, 2, 6, 18, 39, 49–51, 58
Cortiocotrophin releasing factor (CRF), 8, 18, 38, 49–51
Cortisol (hydrocortisone), 2, 6, 18, 39, 49–51, 58, 60
CRF (corticotrophin releasing factor), 8, 18, 38, 49–51

Defaecation, 46 ff
Depolarisation, 21
Dickinson, 61
Disturbance detectors, 11 ff, 25 ff, 35, 55
Dog, 33–34
Ductless glands, 5–6

Ears, 4
Effectors, 40 ff, 55, 56, 59, 60, 67
Eggs, 22
Endocrine system, 4, 6, 18
Energy, 1
Epinephrine (adrenaline), 39, 44, 51, 58, 59, 60
Evolution, 40, 45
Exercise, 13, 15, 16, 18, 30, 39, 54
Eyes, 4, 57

Fats, 1, 35
Feedback mechanisms, 17 ff
  negative, 17 ff
  positive, 17, 19 ff
Fever, 48 ff

68

Principles of biological control

Food, 34

Glucagon, 6, 39
Glucose, 1, 4, 6, 38–39
Goldblatt, 65
Gonadotrophin hormones, 6, 22
Growth hormone (somatotrophin), 6, 39
Gut, 4, 6, 34–35, 38

Heart, 7, 15, 43, 57, 58
Heat loss, 11 ff, 18, 25 ff, 37, 49
  production, 11 ff, 18, 25 ff, 37, 149
  sources, 9, 25 ff, 37
Homeostasis, 4 ff
Hormones, 4 ff, 53, 56
Hunger, 33–36
Hunting, 9
Hydrocortisone (cortisol), 2, 6, 18, 39, 49–51, 58, 66
Hypertension, 57 ff
  renal, 58 ff
Hypothalamus, 6–8, 18, 28, 33, 35, 38, 48, 49–51

Impulse, nerve, 21.
Insulin, 6, 39
Islets of Langerhans, 6

Joint receptors, 5, 32–33, 55

Kidneys, 4, 6, 35, 57 ff, 65 ff

Large bowel, 46 ff
Leucocytes, 48, 49
LH (luteinising hormone), 22
LH releasing factor (LRF), 22
Liver, 4
LRF (LH releasing factor), 22
LTH (Luteotrophic hormone, prolactin), 6
Lungs, 13, 15

Mathematics, 25
Membrane potential, 20, 21
Mid-West, 37
Milk, 6
Misalignment detectors, 12 ff, 25 ff, 35, 54
Muscle, 5, 15, 30–32, 39, 46, 51, 52

Negative feedback, 17 ff
Nerve impulse, 20, 21
Nitrites, 53
Noradrenaline (norepinephrine), 58, 59, 60
Norepinephrine (noradrenaline), 58, 59, 60

Oesophageal fistula, 34
Ovaries, 6, 22
Ovulation, 22–23
Oxygen, 1, 4

Pancreas, 6, 39
Paraplegics, 46
Parathyroids, 8, 55
Phaeochromocytoma, 58, 59
Pituitary, 6 ff, 39
  anterior, 6, 18, 22, 38
  posterior, 6
Positive feedback, 17, 19 ff
Potential difference, 20
Potential, resting, 20
Progesterone, 22
Prolactin, 6
Pyrogen, 48, 49

Receptors, sensory, 4 ff, 35, 41, 46 ff, 53 ff, 60, 61, 62, 67
Releasing factors, 7–8
Renal artery clamps, 65
Renal hypertension, 65 ff
Renin, 65 ff
Resistance, of blood vessels, 43 ff, 58 ff
Resting membrane potential, 20

69